Auditory Neuropathy:

A New Perspective on

Hearing Disorders

Auditory Neuropathy: A New Perspective on Hearing Disorders

Edited by

Yvonne Sininger, Ph.D.

Director, Children's Auditory Research and Evaluation Center
House Ear Institute
Los Angeles, California

Arnold Starr, M.D.

Professor of Neurology
University of California, Irvine
Irvine, California

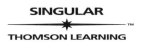

SINGULAR

™

THOMSON LEARNING

Australia   Canada   Mexico   Singapore   Spain   United Kingdom   United States

SINGULAR

THOMSON LEARNING ™

Auditory Neuropathy: A New Perspective on Hearing Disorders
Edited by Yvonne Sininger, Ph.D., and Arnold Starr, M.D.

Business Unit Director: William Brottmiller	**Executive Marketing Manager:** Dawn Gerrain	**Executive Production Editor:** Barb Bullock
Acquisitions Editor: Marie Linvill	**Channel Manager:** Tara Carter	**Production Editor:** Brad Bielawski
Editorial Assistant: Cara Jenkins		

COPYRIGHT © 2001 by Singular, an imprint of Delmar, a division of Thomson Learning, Inc.
Thomson Learning™ is a trademark used herein under license

Printed in Canada
1 2 3 4 5 XXX 06 05 04 02 01

For more information contact Singular,
401 West "A" Street, Suite 325
San Diego, CA 92101-7904
Or find us on the World Wide Web at http://www.singpub.com

For permission to use material from this text or product, contact us by
Tel (800) 730-2214
Fax (800) 730-2215
www.thomsonrights.com

Library of Congress Cataloging-in-Publication Data
Auditory neuropathy : a new perspective on hearing disorders / edited by Yvonne Sininger, Arnold Starr.
    p. ; cm.
  Includes bibliographical references and index.
  ISBN 0-7693-0046-4 (alk. paper)
  1. Hearing disorders.
2. Cochlea—Pathophysiology.
I. Sininger, Yvonne. II. Starr, Arnold, Ph.D.
  [DNLM: 1. Hearing Disorders. 2. Cochlear Nerve—physiopathology. WV 270 A9164 2001]
RF291.A945 2001
617.8—dc21
                            00-049239

NOTICE TO THE READER

Contents

Preface

Arnold Starr and Yvonne Sininger

Early in 1987 I received a call from Dr. Yvonne Sininger at the House Ear Institute asking if I would help evaluate a child of 9 years of age with inconsistent measures of pure tone hearing and "funny looking" ABRs. I accepted, of course, because I learn the most from patients with symptoms and test results that are baffling. The child who we will call "Eve" was 8 years old when she began to have difficulties following her teacher's instructions. She was moved to the front row in school but to no avail. An audiogram showed only a mild-to-moderate sensitivity loss, whereas speech comprehension was disproportionately affected. The ABR was not normal and was interpreted as being either absent or containing short latency components (waves I, II, and III) reflecting activity in the 8th nerve and cochlear nucleus.

Eve and her family came to my laboratory at the University of California early in 1987, and we recorded her auditory evoked potentials. We used rarefaction click signals of 75 dB nHL, which Eve could clearly hear. The ABRs showed short-latency components between 0.5 to 3 ms after stimulus onset, no wave V, and middle and long-latency components were also absent. The child could clearly hear the signals used for testing, but the averaged evoked potentials from auditory nerve to auditory cortex were absent. The bases for this paradox occupied my thoughts for the next year, and Eve and her family worked closely with us (myself, David McPherson, Julie Patterson at Irvine, and Yvonne Sininger, Manny Don, Lisa Tonakawa, Bill Luxford, Mickey Waring, and Bob Shannon at the House Ear Institute in Los Angeles) to understand Eve's dilemma.

Several important "Ahas" occurred that led to the interpretation that the disorder of hearing reflected altered temporal processing of the auditory nerve in the presence of normal cochlear hair cell function.

First, the short latency ABR components that we and others found were actually cochlear microphonics reflecting activity of the hair cells, but no neural components of the ABR were present. Later, we were also able to use the newly described method known as otoacoustic emissions to define that OAEs were also present in Eve. Thus, the cochlea seemed to be normal yet no auditory pathway evoked activity could be defined beginning with the 8th nerve. Eve could hear but the brain was silent. Why?

Second, measures of Eve's hearing capacity provided insight into which aspects of auditory processing were *especially* affected. The tests revealed *marked* deficits in tasks requiring temporal cues: elevation of the time required to distinguish two clicks from one, abnormally large amounts of time needed to detect a silent gap in an auditory signal, inability to localize sounds, failure to detect binaural beats, and absence of masking level differences (MLD). Eve had disordered temporal processing. The extent of the temporal processing deficits was out-of-proportion to the degree of the pure-tone loss and beyond those that accompany hearing loss associated with cochlear receptor hair cell damage.

We formulated Eve's disorder as an alteration of the temporal encoding or synchrony of discharge occurring at the level of the auditory nerve accounting for both the psychoacoustic deficits and the inability to define averaged evoked potentials. We speculated that the deficit might be at the synapse between the inner hair cells and auditory nerve dendrites because the neurological exam was normal without evidence of other cranial nerve or peripheral nerve involvements.

Our manuscript describing Eve was submitted to the journal *Brain* in 1989 and eventually accepted for publication in 1991. This journal has a tradition of publishing results from individual cases that might provide insights into clinical neurological disorders.

We thought we would never see another patient like Eve.

In 1993, Dr. Charles (Chuck) Berlin in New Orleans described several patients with absent ABRs, preserved OAEs, and hearing loss; the constellation of findings seemed similar to those found in Eve. Dr. Terry Picton in Toronto encountered a similar patient. Chuck suggested that Terry and I come to New Orleans to meet and think about this disorder. We jumped at the opportunity and sat together one morning at the Kresge Hearing Center in New Orleans considering the sites and mechanisms in the auditory periphery that could be affected in the disorder. Our short list included (a) inner hair cells, (b) the synapse between the inner hair cells and the auditory nerve dendrites, and (c) the auditory nerve. All seemed likely but difficult to separate from each other by the clinical methods and tests we had available.

We interviewed several of the New Orleans patients and the patient from Toronto to determine if their insights into the hearing loss might be of help. One of Dr. Berlin's patients had a slight clumsiness when she walked into the room. I asked Chuck if he could obtain a reflex hammer, a 128 Hz tuning fork, and an opthalmoscope from the clinic so I could do a brief neurological exam on this patient. There was absence of deep tendon reflexes at the ankles, elevated thresholds for appreciation of vibration in the toes, and a gait ataxia. These findings elicited a big "Aha" as we now had evidence that this new type of hearing disorder could be accompanied by a peripheral neuropathy. Two more patients seen that day also had a peripheral neuropathy. The designation "auditory neuropathy" seemed appropriate for the disorder. A second paper authored by myself and Sininger from California, Picton from Canada, and Berlin and Dr. Linda Hood from New Orleans describing 10 patients, 7 of whom had a peripheral neuropathy, was published in *Brain* in 1996.

By 1998, interest in this disorder was growing rapidly as others around the country and the world were seeing patients with this constellation of symptoms and wondering about the physiology and prognosis and how to proceed with intervention. In March of that year, supported by the National Institute of Deafness and Other Communicative Disorders, we invited a group of experts to contribute to a meeting of minds to share information and brainstorm about auditory neuropathy. The authors in this volume are some of those who contributed to that conference at Lake Arrowhead, California. They have provided complete descriptions demonstrating the variety of findings and symptoms of patients that fall under the category of auditory neuropathy, information about the criteria for diagnosis, the prevalence of this disorder in newborns, the type and extent of hearing loss, details of the psychophysics of the hearing loss, the role of efferents in this disorder, the pathology of the temporal bone, the neurology and pathophysiology of the disorder, and the effectiveness of rehabilitation including the use of cochlear implants and hearing aids.

As clinicians and scientists, it is important to listen to our patients for insight into the nature of any disorder. Much was learned about the nature of auditory neuropathy from careful study of Eve. She is now in her early twenties and has recently received a cochlear implant. These are her insights into her disorder, just prior to being implanted:

WALKING THROUGH THE LIFE

OF AN *UNSURE* GIRL

Hearing, but never comprehending

What is that? A sound she hears? What is THAT sound in the distance? That "one" you *know*? Is it *really* a sound she wonders, or merely a humbug in her head?

Sound here. . . .
Sound there. . . .

No meaning. . . . Just "sounds."

Annoying sounds. . . .

GO A-W-A-Y!!

These *sounds* keep her mind racing 24 hours a day.

Seeking
so
desperately
to
underSTAND

The calls, the bangs, the thumps, the beats. . . .

HEARING

FEELING

But never *truly* comprehending.

This is the girl, who so desperately wants to understand, she forces her mind to constantly "go"—always on the look-out for cues, in hopes she may for one moment in time,

Comprehend.

No time to rest the body, the soul—for the *sounds* she hears, have become her biggest enemy, constantly fighting, but never winning.

We conclude with an excerpt from an adult, male patient who we will call Adam (not his real name). Adam has a moderate-to-mild, low-frequency hearing loss with nearly normal thresholds at 2000 Hz and above. He has an ABR with very poor waveform morphology including a poorly formed, low-amplitude wave V, but clear evidence of cochlear microphonic and normal otoacoustic emissions. He describes some of his experiences living with auditory neuropathy. It is noteworthy that his hearing appears to have been normal until adolescence, and his language and speech skills are very good.

Adam is a handsome, gregarious, successful engineer who is frustrated by professionals who do not understand his situation and especially by not being able to speak on the phone. His speechreading skills are exceptional and, consequently, the extent of his communication impairment is often underestimated and misunderstood. Here is his situation in his own words.

My name is . . . . I have a nerve disorder that impairs my ability to understand speech and hear some sounds. Please look at me and communicate your thoughts effectively, and it helps to let me know the subject matter and when you plan on changing it. Also, if I respond unintelligently to your question, it's because I misunderstood you. As you can see I am quite confident that if I hear what you are saying, I'll respond with a piece of genius wit!

When I was asked to write a few words on what it is like to live with auditory neuropathy, I began to think of my past experiences and the chronology of attempts to solve this problem. One of the most frustrating aspects of my journey thus far is the enigma surrounding the type of hearing loss I have. The nature of the hearing problem I have is very puzzling to me as well as to my friends and family. I seem to hear sounds and noises just fine, but it is extremely difficult for me to comprehend the speech of others.

My life as a young boy was very normal; I grew up in a large family. I have four, very loud sisters; I am the only boy. Maybe the hearing problem was sent as a gift! As far as my family and I know, I did not have a hearing impairment until adolescence. I did have an audiogram as part of a physical when I was 10 years old; the results were normal. At the pubescent age of 15 I began to notice that I was having problems understanding what people were saying. As we all know, at the age of 16, boys need to be boys; not being able to ask a girl out on the phone, or respond to another boy's wise cracks, was a big issue.

I also noticed that when other people would hear low-tone sounds, I was not able to hear the sound. I went to an audiologist and received an examination. The test showed a "reverse slope hearing loss." The hearing aid distributor assured me that this would not be a problem to "fix." Many years and dollars later, I never felt that the hearing aids helped me. To make a long story short, a miracle never transpired.

One positive aspect of wearing hearing aids was the fact that other people noticed the hearing aids, made the inference that I had a hearing problem and, as a result, made an effort speak while facing me. In addition, the hearing aid was an automatic explanation to people when I did not hear them. This "placebo" effect of the hearing aids was not enough to offset the discomfort the aids caused; as a result, I never wore them for any substantial period of time. The fact that I did not want to wear the aids led people to believe that I was just too vain to wear them; they didn't seem to believe me when I explained to them that the hearing aids were not helping my situation.

My university years were filled with fun times and success despite my hearing problem. I attended a large public university and received a degree in civil engineering without the use of note takers or any special accommodations. In fact, only a few of my past teachers were aware of my hearing loss/impairment. Socially, I experienced great success. I was an active member of a large fraternity. I was very involved in social functions and participated on a number of college committees.

If you asked me what I liked most about myself, I would say the number and quality of friends I share. In addition to friendships, I was able to meet and marry the woman of my dreams. Not too shabby for a guy who has only 20-40% speech comprehension.

I did experience many uncomfortable situations and obstacles due to my hearing loss. For the most part, I was able to find a way to communicate through other means. I don't think I can put my finger on the exact definition of "other means" but I'm guessing it's a mixture of reading lips, body language, and analyzing a little mental matrix of possible words. I have never taken a lip-reading class; every technique that I use has come from natural adaptation.

Telephone conversations are very difficult for me, as well as hearing any speech from any source other than a person looking directly at me. It is virtually impossible for me to follow a radio talk show, but I do listen to music often.

I like music and I love to dance, but it's entertaining to hear me sing the words that I think the musician is singing. Most of the time, after being corrected, I conclude that the wrong lyrics sound better and make more sense. I seem to hear high tones exceptionally well; I can hear my neighbor's phone ringing when my wife can't. I am usually the first to notice a high pitch sound, but the last to know if it's there is a low tone sound.

After graduation I began a career in engineering and I have excelled in the technical aspects of my work, which has rewarded me with many promotions and job opportunities. With each promotion, the need to communicate on the phone and in meetings with several people was greater. I began to realize that I must do something if I wanted to continue upward mobility.

Out of desperation, I set out to give hearing aids another try, hoping that maybe the technology was there now. After going through a similar experience as before, I was ready to give up on pursuing any type of treatment. I decided to try one more doctor before I gave up on the audiologist for good.

I flipped through a phone book randomly and set another appointment; this time the doctor had a hunch when I was not responding to the hearing aids. To make a long story short, I have been diagnosed with auditory neuropathy. The explanation of this disorder has helped me understand why I do not understand speech as well as I should. I also feel that being diagnosed with this disorder has justified the fact that the hearing aids did not work.

Where to go from here is the next question I have. For now I will have to settle for what this society has provided for hearing-impaired people. Having explored almost every available special accommodation for the hearing impaired, I have been very disappointed by the technology and accessibility provided to our hearing-impaired patrons. My long list of complaints begins with the dazzling 1960s techno wonder called TTY and continues with the fact that hearing aids are not covered by most insurance policies. No movie theaters have closed captioning available; also it really makes me mad when I can't understand important messages over the PA system at airports.

I'll step off my soapbox now, and say this; hearing 100% is not necessary in order to lead a joyful and contributing life. But it would be nice to have a "miracle" so I can pursue life with out the worry that I might not understand what you, or more importantly, my children are saying.

Those of us with normal hearing (or even those with more typical, sensory hearing loss for that matter) will never truly comprehend the acoustic events perceived (or misperceived) by persons suffering from auditory neuropathy, because we cannot hear the world through their ears. The previous passages, taken directly from adults with this disorder, shed some important insight into their auditory worlds for researchers, clinicians, and lay persons who come in contact with them and who share an interest in diagnosing, understanding, and helping to relieve their disorder. We believe that listening to insights of these adult patients who can describe their auditory sensations will help us to understand how to help those very young children with auditory neuropathy who are struggling to use their hearing to learn speech and language, and we appreciate their candor.

The editors of this volume are also grateful and acknowledge the support of the National Institute of Deafness and Other Communicative Disorders for their support of the Conference on Auditory Neuropathy and for our research, much of which is highlighted in this text.

Dedication

Dr. Laszlo Stein,
Professor of Otolaryngology, Head & Neck Surgery
Professor of Audiology and Hearing Science
Northwestern University

This volume is dedicated to the memory of our esteemed colleague and friend, Laszlo Stein. His contribution to our understanding of auditory neuropathy and of all areas of auditory dysfunction in infants and children from special populations was vast. Throughout his long and productive career, Dr. Stein focused on the needs of children with hearing loss. He was a pioneer in the area of assessment, developing clinical skills and research protocols in electrophysiology that allowed him to provide diagnostic and rehabilitative services for the most difficult of cases, including newborns and infants and those children with multiple disorders from special populations. Early in his career he served as an Assistant Professor at the Institute for Study of Exceptional Children at DePaul University in Chicago and continued this line of work throughout his lifetime. His first research grant was entitled "Identification and Evaluation of at-Risk Deaf-Blind Children and Youth," followed almost immediately by another called "A Model Project for Hearing-Handicapped Infants Providing Medical, Academic and Psychological Services."

Laszlo was involved at every level of the process of improving the lives of children with special needs and hearing loss. He was a clinician and clinic administrator at the Siegel Institute of Michael Reese Medical Center in Chicago for more than 20 years. He was an author and teacher throughout his career, contributing in such diverse areas as parent counseling and electrophysiologic assessment of hearing and auditory function. He served his fellow professionals in many ways, as a member of many professional organizations, serving on boards and committees. One of his most notable contributions was serving for 10 years as Section Editor for Electrophysiology for the journal *Ear and Hearing*.

Laszlo was a co-author with Nina Kraus and colleagues on a manuscript in 1984 that first described the phenomenon we now call auditory neuropathy. Years later, while working with local hospitals to develop programs for early identification of hearing loss in neonates, Laszlo discovered a group of infants from the newborn intensive care unit who demonstrated severely abnormal auditory brain stem responses but normal otoacoustic emissions. His careful description of these infants led to an understanding of the link between auditory neuropathy and hyperbillirubinemia. At least one of the children identified by Dr. Stein is discussed in this book in Chapter 11 by Trautwein et al. It was Dr. Stein who encouraged me to hold our 1998 Conference on Auditory Neuropathy at Lake Arrowhead where he was a featured speaker discussing high-risk neonates with auditory neuropathy. His influence is seen throughout this manuscript where he is often cited.

Laszlo will long be remembered by his friends and colleagues. He gave of himself continuously and unselfishly, as a teacher, as a clinician, as a scientist, as a fellow-professional, and as a friend. It is with great respect for his family and for his years of important contribution to children and adults with hearing loss that we dedicate this volume to him.

Selected Publications by Laszlo Stein, Ph.D.

Stein, L. K. (1976). An electrophysiological test of infant hearing. *American Annals of the Deaf, June,* 322–326.

Stein, L., & Kraus, N. (1985). Auditory brainstem response measures with multiply handicapped children and adults. In J.T. Jacobson (Ed.), *The auditory brainstem response* (pp. 337–348). San Diego, CA: College-Hill Press.

Stein, L. K., & Kraus, N. (1988). Auditory evoked potentials with special populations. *Seminars in Hearing, 9,* 35–45.

Stein, L. K., Kraus, N., Ozdamar, O., Cartee, C., Jabaley, T., Jeantele, C., & Reed, N. (1987). Hearing loss in an institutionalized mentally retarded population. Identification by auditory brainstem response. *Archives of Otolaryngology, 113,* 32–35.

Stein, L., Tremblay, K., Pasternak, J., Banerjee, S., Lindemann, K., & Kraus, N. (1996). Brainstem abnormalities in neonates with normal otoacoustic emissions. *Seminars in Hearing, 17,* 197–213.

Auditory Neuropathy Contributors

Charles I. Berlin, Ph.D.
Professor and Director
Kresge Hearing Research
  Laboratory
Department of Otolaryngology
Louisiana State University Health
  Sciences Center
New Orleans, Louisiana

Edward Cohn, M.D.
Staff Otolaryngologist
Boys Town National Research
  Hospital
Associate Professor of
  Otolaryngology and Human
  Communication
Creighton University School of
  Medicine
Omaha, Nebraska

Lee Fabry, M.A.
Clinical Audiologist
Mayo Clinic
Rochester, Minnesota

Rick Friedman, M.D., Ph.D.
House Ear Clinic
House Ear Institute
Los Angeles, California

Smita Garde, Ph.D.
University of Southern California
Los Angeles, California

Robert V. Harrison, Ph.D., DSc.
Auditory Science Laboratory
Department of Otolaryngology
Hospital for Children
University of Toronto
Toronto, Ontario
Canada

Linda Hood, Ph.D.
Kresge Hearing Research
  Laboratory
Department of Otolaryngology
Louisiana State University Health
  Sciences Center
New Orleans, Louisiana

Bronya J. Keats, Ph.D.
Professor and Head, Department
  of Genetics
Louisiana State University Health
  Sciences Center
New Orleans, Louisiana

Judith B. Kenyon
Research Technologist II
Center for Human Molecular
  Genetics
Munroe-Meyer Institute
University of Nebraska Medical
  Center
Omaha, Nebraska

Ronald Kim, M.D.
University of California, Irvine
Irvine, California

William Kimberling, Ph.D.
Director, Genetics Department
Boys Town National Research
   Hospital
Omaha, Nebraska

Karin Kirschhofer, M.D.
Department of Otolaryngology
University of Vienna
Austria

Nina Kraus, Ph.D.
Professor, Department of
   Communication Sciences,
   Neurology, Physiology and
   Otolaryngology
Northwestern University
Evanston, Illinois

Fred H. Linthicum Jr., M.D.
Department of Histopathology
House Ear Institute
Los Angeles, California

Jean K. Moore, Ph.D.
Department of Neuroanatomy
House Ear Institute
Los Angeles, California

Joseph B. Nadol, Jr., M.D.
Department of Otology and
   Laryngology
Harvard Medical School
Department of Otolaryngology
Massachusetts Eye and Ear
   Infirmary
Boston, Massachusetts

Sandy Oba, M.S.
Research Audiologist
House Ear Institute
Los Angeles, California

Terence W. Picton, M.D.
Rotman Research Institute
Baycrest Centre for Geriatric Care
Toronto, Ontario
Canada

Gary Rance, MSc.
Department of Otolaryngology
The University of Melbourne
East Melbourne, Victoria
Australia

Renee Rogers, B.A.
Graduate Student
Boys Town National Research
   Hospital
Genetics Department
Omaha, Nebraska

John Shallop, Ph.D.
Audiologist, Mayo Clinic
Rochester, Minnesota

Yvonne S. Sininger, Ph.D.
Director, Children's Auditory
   Research and Evaluation
   Center
House Ear Institute
Los Angeles, California

Arnold Starr, M.D.
Professor of Neurology
University of California, Irvine
Irvine, California

Patricia Glenna Trautwein, M.A.
Pediatric Audiologist
House Ear Institute
Los Angeles, California

Barbara Cone-Wesson, Ph.D.
Department of Otolaryngology
The University of Melbourne
East Melbourne, Victoria
Australia

Fan-Gang Zeng, Ph.D.
Otolaryngology
University of California, Irvine
Irvine, California

Auditory Neuropathy: An Historical and Current Perspective

Nina Kraus

EVOLUTION OF THE CONCEPT

It was almost 20 years ago that audiologists began to hear about patients with absent auditory brain stem responses (ABRs), but normal or near-normal audiograms. In the early 1980s, Davis and Hirsh (1979), Worthington and Peters (1980), and Lenhardt (1981) were among the first to publish case accounts of people with absent ABRs and normal or near-normal hearing thresholds.

Kraus Özdamar, Stein, and Reed (1984) reported on 3 years of accumulated clinical data. Of 543 children with no clinical evidence of brain stem damage evaluated for "suspected hearing loss," 49 had absent ABRs. Most of these patients had audiometrically confirmed severe-to-profound hearing loss, whereas 7 had audiograms showing no worse than a moderate hearing loss. That is, 14% of "absent ABR" cases, and 1.3% of the total population evaluated for hearing loss, had evidence of this combination of results. Davis and Hirsh (1979) reported a smaller but significant incidence in their clinic population: 1 in 200 or 0.5%. Berlin and colleagues reported auditory neuropathy in 5 of 60 (12%) children diagnosed as "deaf" (1994, 1998). Thus, early estimates ranged from .5 to 1.3% of the clinical population and 12 to 14% of those who would otherwise have been thought to have a severe-to-profound cochlear hearing loss.

Initially, the notion of an absent ABR with normal or only mildly impaired audiometric thresholds met with considerable skepticism—not only in the peer-reviewed literature, but also in the clinic. The appeal to

1

technical error was frequent. More important, children's parents were confused. The definitive test (ABR) indicated deafness, but the children displayed behavioral responses to sound. A hallmark of the condition is inconsistent response to sound, and this complicated delineation of the condition. With children, the inconsistency could be due to less than optimal cooperation and motivation. Furthermore, because the vast majority of patients with absent ABR have cochlear pathology when faced with a poor ABR result, most clinicians assumed that patients had conventional hearing loss and discounted inconsistent responses to sound. The result was that auditory neuropathy patients were subject to misdiagnosis and incorrect treatment.

Fortunately, understanding and awareness of this pattern of results have improved. The addition of otoacoustic emissions (OAEs) to the testing repertoire has helped to refine our assessment (Gravel, Kurtzberg, Stapells, Vaughn, & Wallace, 1989; Norton, 1993; Prieve, Gorga, & Neely, 1991; Vohr, White, & Maxon Johnson, 1993). Particularly important have been the persistent efforts by Starr, Sininger, Berlin, Picton, Stein and others in informing the clinical and research communities of the condition (Berlin, 1996; Berlin & Hood 1993; Berlin et al., 1993; Picton, 1986; Picton et al., 1981; Sininger, Hood, Starr, Berlin, & Picton, 1995; Starr et al., 1991, 1998, 1995; Starr, Picton, Sininger, Hood, & Berlin, 1996; Stein et al., 1996). Figure 1–1 charts the numbers of papers about auditory neuropathy that have been published over the past 20 years. Roughly 50 papers have been published to date, and as is evident from the graph, the number of published reports is rising. The papers were categorized as to whether they were case reports or reports that addressed mechanisms underlying auditory neuropathy. There has been an increasing interest in discovering underlying anatomic and physiologic processes. Overall, these cases have provided clinical challenges for diagnosis and treatment. More theoretically, they have challenged our thinking about the physiology of hearing— and specifically about our ability to provide a model for examining the role of neural synchrony of the 8th nerve and brain stem on perception.

In these 20 years, this constellation of results has been given a variety of names, including *paradoxical, brain stem auditory processing syndrome* (BAPS), *central auditory dysfunction,* and *neural synchrony disorder.* Most recently, researchers and clinicians have proffered and accepted the term *auditory neuropathy,* although whether the condition is, in fact, a neuropathy is not yet established.

A clinical definition of auditory neuropathy has emerged. By definition, patients with this disorder have normal otoacoustic emissions (OAEs) and cochlear microphonic (CM), but an absent or severely abnormal ABR. Other clinical characteristics appear to vary. Tone thresholds can range from normal or near-normal sensitivity to severe impairment. Impaired auditory processing skills typically are reported, especially in noisy

Auditory Neuropathy Publications by Year
1979 - present

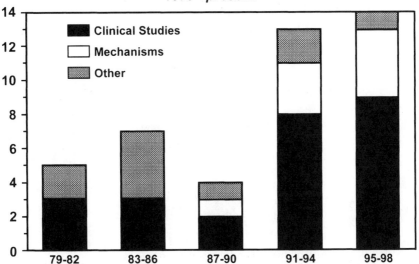

Figure 1–1. The number of papers concerning auditory neuropathy published over the past 20 years. The papers (detailed in the reference list) were categorized as to whether they were case reports or studies that addressed mechanisms underlying auditory neuropathy. There has been an increasing interest in discovering underlying anatomic and physiologic processes.

environments. Acoustic reflexes are absent. Some cases are transient or intermittent; others change little over time and may even worsen.

CLINICAL SYMPTOMATOLOGY AND AUDITORY PATHWAY ETIOLOGIES

It is important to establish which factors predispose a child to auditory neuropathy, yet this, too, turns out to be a difficult issue. Auditory neuropathy can occur in the absence of any apparent medical problem, or it can be associated with a variety of other symptoms and conditions (Table 1–1), such as infectious processes (e.g., mumps), immune disorders, and various genetic and syndromal conditions (e.g., mitochondrial enzymatic deficit, Freidreich's ataxia, Stevens-Johnson syndrome, Ehrlers-Danlos syndrome, and Charcot-Marie-Tooth syndrome; Cassandro et al., 1986; Deltenre et al., 1997; Ferber-Viart et al., 1994; Hardin, 1995; Kalaydjieva et al., 1996; Nelson et al., 1988; Satya-Murti et al., 1983: Sawada, 1979).

Table 1–1. Medical conditions encompassed by the auditory neuropathy umbrella.

Unremarkable medical history

Anoxia

Hyperbilirubinemia

Infectious processes (e.g., mumps)

Immune disorders (e.g., Guillain-Barre syndrome)

Genetic and syndromal
    Hereditary sensory motor neuropathy
    Mitochondrial enzymatic deficit
    Olivo-pontine-cerebellar degeneration
    Freidreich's ataxia
    Stevens-Johnson syndrome
    Ehrlers-Danlos syndrome
    Charcot-Marie-Tooth syndrome

Permanent (all of the above)

Transient (hyperbilirubinemia, anoxia)

Intermittent (fever)

It also has been shown to occur with diffuse neonatal insults such as anoxia, hyperbilirubinemia, and acidosis (Chisin et al., 1979; Deltenre et al., 1997; Kraus et al., 1984; Silver et al., 1995; Stein et al., 1996), as well as transiently with fever (Gorga et al., 1995; Starr et al., 1998). The heterogeneity of the population thus makes it a great challenge to diagnose, understand, and treat these individuals.

Of great interest are the possible physiologic underpinnings of these test results. Based on symptomatology and the known generation sites of ABRs and OAEs, various possible anatomic and physiologic bases for dysfunction have been proposed, including the cochlea, brain stem, and almost anything in between. Harrison (1988) emphasized the electrical–mechanical transduction processes of inner hair cells (see also Schrott, Stephan, & Speondlin, 1989). Chisin et al. (1979) and more recently Starr et al. (1996) emphasized the axons, cell bodies, and myelin sheath of the auditory nerve (hence, "auditory neuropathy"). The auditory brain stem pathway has been a suspect (Gorga et al., 1995; Kraus et al., 1984) and has been particularly implicated in cases of bilirubinemia (Barbary 1991a, 1991b; Gupta et al., 1990; Nakamura et al., 1985; Shapiro, 1994; Stein et al., 1996). Gravel and Stapells (1993) cited a combination of peripheral and central pathways. Hienz, Stiles, and May (1998) suggested efferent influences (olivocochlear feedback). That so many sites serve as suspects suggests that auditory neuropathy encompasses a variety of disorders sharing in common the symptom that OAEs are present and ABRs are dramatically abnormal. As such, it is a neural synchrony disorder.

TREATMENT CONSIDERATIONS

Another issue of great interest is that of treatment and management of patients. Can hearing aids help a child who appears to have near normal thresholds? Will the pulsatile stimulation of auditory nerve fibers via a cochlear implant be a better mode of stimulation for central pathways than the deficient neural response that characterizes auditory neuropathy? Will rehabilitative training be of use, and if so, what type(s) of training? Will speech-sound training be best, or must auditory cues be combined with visual cues, as in cued speech, lipreading, or even sign language?

More questions than answers surround the issue of treatment of auditory neuropathy. Treatment has not been considered systematically. Many audiologists have the impression that hearing aids cannot help, that amplification may hinder perception, and that higher intensities of sound may damage an apparently intact cochlea. The hearing aid issue is not straightforward because many patients have elevated thresholds that might be improved by amplification, and there have been reports of benefit from hearing aids and FM systems in some patients. On the other hand, there have been a few reports of loss of OAEs following hearing aid use, and the correct approach is not clear at this time. The prevailing treatment seems to be conservative trials with amplification devices, with diligent monitoring of amplification output levels and otoacoustic emissions, and utmost consideration of patient and parent feedback regarding benefits (see the Cone-Wesson, Rance, & Sininger Chapter 12 in this text on rehabilitation for details).

Might electrical stimulation help in some cases? Several reports have indicated that electrical stimulation is effective in providing useful auditory information for speech perception (Sininger et al., 1999; Trautwein et al., 2000). Information and discussion on several cases of children with auditory neuropathy who have received cochlear implantation can be found in this volume in Chapter 12 by Trautwein, Shallop, Fabry, and Friedman.

Directed perceptual training may be a possible option. Speech-sound training has been shown to modify perception in other populations. For example, people can be trained to hear sounds that do not occur in their native language (Bradlow, 1997; Pisoni et al., 1982). Speech-sound training can also help children with perceptually based learning problems (Ball & Blachman, 1991; Bradley & Bryant, 1983; Byrne & Fielding-Barnsley, 1993; Lundberg et al., 1988; Merzenich et al., 1996; Shankweiler at al., 1995;

Tallal et al., 1996). From a physiologic standpoint, training-associated reorganization has been demonstrated primarily at higher levels of the auditory pathway, particularly auditory thalamus and cortex in experimental animals (Buchwald et al., 1966; Harrison et al., 1993; Kraus & Disterhoft, 1982; Merzenich et al., 1991; Reale et al., 1987; Recanzone et al., 1993; Robertson & Irvine 1989; Weinberger et al., 1984). In humans, less is known about plasticity at lower levels of the system and the extent to which cortical receptive fields can be modified to make the most use of the impoverished information that does make it through the system (Gatehouse, 1992; Kraus et al., 1995; Naatanen, 1993; Neville et al., 1983; Tremblay et al., 1997; 1998). Also to be established is the content of such training (i.e., determining what are the essential acoustic elements to train).

Might formal training with visual cues help? There is a strong scientific basis for the notion that visual input can enhance and alter auditory perception. For example, visual information from speech-like lip movements has been shown to modify auditory cortex activity (Sams et al., 1991). Physiologic changes in auditory cortex can occur during lipreading, even in the absence of auditory stimulation (Calvert et al., 1997). Therefore, the intact visual modality might be used to enhance auditory perception—"to hear with one's eyes."

IMPACT ON SPEECH PERCEPTION

A key issue is the effect of auditory neuropathy on speech perception. Even with near-normal thresholds, auditory neuropathy significantly affects speech perception, with reports ranging from functionally deaf to relatively intact speech perception in quiet with severely impaired perception in noise. It is not known whether perceptual impairments lie on a continuum or whether the nature of the impairment differs qualitatively from patient to patient. Our understanding of the perceptual consequences has been complicated because most cases have co-occurring elevated hearing thresholds, making it is difficult to disentangle the effects of audibility and the neuropathy.

Also limiting our understanding of speech perception with auditory neuropathy is that as clinicians and scientists, we are just beginning to think about what measures are likely to provide the most insight into the perceptual deficits and strengths that have the greatest bearing on speech perception ability in natural communication settings. An in-depth understanding of the specific perceptual deficits associated with auditory neuropathy requires a detailed approach. One such report of psychophysical abilities in an individual with auditory neuropathy was provided by Starr and colleagues (1991). That report is summarized here, along with another case that was evaluated according to a combined behavioral–neurophysiologic, acoustic–phonetic approach that we have applied to various investigations of biologic processes involved in speech-sound perception. This experimental approach examines the relationship among listeners' perception of acoustic signals, the neurophysiologic representation of those same signals, and other behavioral measures of speech perception and language processing in order to link perception of speech to underlying central physiological processes (Carrell et al., 1999; Koch et al., 1999; Kraus et al., 1996, 1999).

Starr et al. (1991) described a series of classic psychophysical measures obtained from an adolescent with auditory neuropathy. Temporal processing deficits were evident. Gap detection was poor (i.e., 100 ms vs. the normal 2-ms threshold). Binaural signal processing for both time and intensity cues was impaired, and the patient had no masking level differences with dichotic inversions of phase, another indication of impaired binaural processing. Frequency and intensity discrimination to pure tones was impaired, with the patient requiring 3 to 15 times the normal frequency change and twice the normal intensity change to discriminate differences. Despite these deficits, the patient demonstrated relatively normal trade-off of stimulus intensity and duration, a function that is typically impaired in patients with cochlear damage. How these impaired psychoacoustic abilities relate to speech perception was not addressed by Starr and colleagues but is covered in detail in Chapter 8 by Zeng, Oba, Garde, Sininger, and Starr in this volume.

In another case, described in detail by Kraus et al. (1993, 2000), speech perception was studied in a young woman (IT) with auditory neuropathy. Her case is particularly instructive because she has no coincident audiometric hearing loss, thus, it is possible to evaluate the consequences of neural asynchrony without the complication of having to disentangle the effects of audibility. Moreover, the patient is a bright, cooperative young adult who has good insight into her condition. Her profile may provide a "best-case scenario" of how well a person with absent ABRs and present OAEs may function.

IT is a young adult with a largely unremarkable medical history and normal intellectual and academic performance based on standardized tests. Throughout her childhood, hearing tests indicated a normal audiogram and therefore her auditory symptoms were dismissed. As an adult, she reports that she is "deaf " in noisy environments, although she reports little or no difficulty in ideal listening situations.

IT has a normal audiogram, absent ABR, absent acoustic reflexes, and normal distortion product otoacoustic emissions. Formal testing of open-set word and sentence recognition in quiet indicated good speech perception (Luce & Pisoni, 1988; CUNY Sentences, auditory only). However, speech perception was deficient when fine-grained perception was assessed. Discrimination thresholds for synthetic CV syllables (fine-grained differences of speech sound structure in quiet) suggested difficulty discriminating stimuli that differ in spectrotemporal characteristics at stimulus onset, but no difficulty discriminating stimuli that differ in the temporal domain (see Kraus et al., 1999, and Carrell et al., 1999 for description of stimuli, experimental procedures, and normative data). This pattern is not unlike that observed in certain children with learning problems (Kraus et al., 1996). Similar to behavioral testing in quiet, evoked responses reflecting activity of pathways central to the brain stem (i.e., middle latency responses, P1N1, mismatch negativity [MMN], and P300 cortical responses) were largely intact, with abnormalities observed only when responses reflected neural representation of fine-grained acoustic–phonetic elements.

Despite the fact that poor speech perception in noise is the hallmark impairment reported by every case with the diagnosis of auditory neuropathy, little formal data exist. In noise, IT's perception was markedly impaired to the aforementioned open-set word recognition measures. Specifically, for IT a drop of 25% correct occurred from +12 signal-to-noise ratio (SNR) to +9 SNR, whereas normal subjects showed little change in these SNR conditions. At +3 SNR, IT was severely impaired, getting only 10% correct compared with the normal-hearing subjects who still got almost 50% correct.

Like normal-hearing subjects, lexical difficulty affected IT's word recognition (Luce & Pisoni, 1998), and she was able to make use of consistent talker information provided by a single talker compared with constantly changing talker information in a multiple-talker condition. This suggests that, even in noise, she is sensitive to the nonlinguistic, qualitative aspects of the signal and is able to adapt to a particular speaking style. In addition, IT follows the normal pattern of discriminating phonemes: final consonants were most prone to error, vowels were resistant to error, and place of articulation was most vulnerable.

This case illustrates the extent to which speech perception can be preserved and how it is impaired when neural synchrony is disrupted. In quiet, only fine-grained speech perception was impaired. In noise, IT followed the same pattern of perceptual impairment and phonetic confusions seen in normal subjects, but the deficits were extraordinarily exaggerated. Thus, excellent speech perception is possible with absent ABR. That is, the ABR may be quite sensitive to timing and synchrony disruption as evidenced by absent peaks in the waveform, but disruption of 8th nerve and auditory brain stem synchrony may not impair understanding of speech in ideal listening situations. On the other hand, an intact ABR appears to indicate that synchrony makes an important difference when listening in the presence of noise, which is what we do most of the time. It is also apparent that the central pathways can make use of varied and limited input that can be interpreted as speech by the brain.

Of course, these deficits and strengths should not be construed as a characterization of all patients with absent ABRs and present OAEs, some of which demonstrate considerable amounts of hearing loss and poor speech perception in quiet, but they do raise interesting questions and serve as a model for the characterization of subsequent patients. Effective assessment measures will need to be delineated and developed on a much larger sample of subjects such that the wide range of perceptual abilities evident in patients with auditory neuropathy can be understood.

SUMMARY AND FUTURE DIRECTIONS

Despite continuing controversies surrounding auditory neuropathy, we have made progress and learned a great deal since the enigma first surfaced two decades ago. There is now an awareness and acceptance by clinical and research communities that such a disorder indeed exists. The disorder has a name (auditory neuropathy) that facilitates the discussion of the issues. The constellation of symptoms has been described: auditory perception deficits, the varieties of audiometric results, absence or severe abnormality of ABR, absence of acoustic reflexes, and present OAEs. With acceptance and awareness, misdiagnosis is becoming less common, and clinicians have been able to provide what comfort there is in reassuring patients that their complaints are objectively definable.

In addition, the ability to identify the symptomatology has improved. Otoacoustic emissions have provided a measure of cochlear function. Clinicians now routinely distinguish cochlear (CM) from neural (ABR) responses by manipulating click polarity and observing the distinguishing effects of stimulus rate and intensity on response latency. Furthermore, the recent emphasis on neonatal screening programs can result in earlier identification of auditory neuropathy, when both OAEs and ABRs are tested.

Many pieces of information are missing, and we need to develop new tests to fill in our knowledge. Current electrophysiologic tests (i.e., ABR, OAE) provide information about underlying physiologic mechanisms. As-yet-undeveloped measures of neural synchrony, IHC function, and efferent function could increase our understanding of these mechanisms. The extent to which the electrophysiology may provide information about functional capabilities and prognosis remains to be determined.

Behavioral and neurophysiologic testing of fine-grained perception of acoustically well-controlled sounds in quiet and in noise is likely to reveal information about the physiologic mechanisms and functional capabilities, but probably not the prognosis of patients with auditory neuropathy. Formal assessment of speech perception in quiet and in noise, as well as language development and patient and parent reports, should tell us about functional capabilities and prognosis. For example, an approach for assessing multiple facets of auditory function as it relates to speech perception has been briefly described above. Moreover, for very young children, we can draw upon the various measures that have been developed for assessment of language development in children with cochlear implants. Information about how auditory neuropathy affects developmental speech and language milestones will eventually be gathered as babies are followed through infancy and childhood. Medical histories and accompanying conditions will provide information about related symptomatology and physiologic mechanisms.

For the future, we want to understand the various physiologic mechanisms that can give rise to this symptomatology. It will be important to understand the functional capabilities experienced by patients with auditory neuropathy and to document their various perceptual deficits and strengths. Coupled with physiologic measures, this condition provides an opportunity for gaining insights into several important questions in auditory neuroscience of a clinical and scientific nature. To be gained are insights into the role of neural synchrony in the neural representation and perception of sound, and information as to what our diagnostic measures tell us about hearing. Neural and perceptual reorganization with treatment of neuropathy is another issue relevant to larger questions of brain plasticity in neuroscience and to specific clinical populations.

Acknowledgment: Supported by National Institute of Health-National Institute on Deafness and Other Communicative Disorders Grant No. RO1-DC01510.

REFERENCES

Ball, E. W., & Blachman, B. A. (1991). Does phoneme awareness training in kindergarten make a difference in early recognition and developmental spelling? *Reading Research Quarterly, 26,* 49–66.

Barbary, A. E. (1991a). Auditory nerve of the normal and jaundiced rat. I. Spontaneous discharge rate and cochlear nerve histology. *Hearing Research, 54,* 75–90.

Barbary, A. E. (1991b). Auditory nerve of the normal and jaundiced rat. II. Frequency selectivity and two-tone rate suppression. *Hearing Research, 54,* 91–104.

Berlin, C. I. (1996). Role of infant hearing screening in health care. *Seminars in Hearing, 17,* 115–124.

Berlin, C., Bordelon, J., St. John, P., Wilensky, M., Hurley, A., Kluka, E., & Hood, L. (1998). Reversing click polarity may uncover auditory neuropathy in infants. *Ear and Hearing, 19,* 37–47.

Berlin, C. I., & Hood, L. J. (1993). Pseudo-central hearing loss: A confusion of central for peripheral hearing loss caused by faulty conditioning techniques and lax criteria. *Seminars in Hearing, 14,* 215–223.

Berlin, C. I., Hood, L. J., Cecola, R. P., Jackson, D., & Szabo, P. (1993). Afferent-efferent disconnection in humans. *Hearing Research, 65,* 40–50.

Berlin, C. I., Hood, L. J., Hurley, A., & Wen, H. (1994). Contralateral suppression of otoacoustic emissions: An index of the function of the medial olivocochlear system. *Otolaryngology Head and Neck Surgery, 110,* 3–21.

Bradley, L., & Bryant, P. E. (1983). Categorizing sounds and learning to read: A causal connection. *Nature, 301,* 419–421.

Bradlow, A. R. (1997). Training Japanese listeners to identify English /r/ and /l/: IV. Some effects of perceptual learning on speech production. *Journal of the Acoustical Society of America, 101,* 2299–2310.

Buchwald, J., Halas, E., & Schramm, S. (1966). Changes in cortical and subcortical unit activity during behavioral conditioning. *Physiology and Behavior, 1,* 11–22.

Byrne, B., & Fielding-Barnsley, R. (1993). Evaluation of a program to teach phonemic awareness to young children: A 1-year follow-up. *Journal of Educational Psychology, 85,* 104–111.

Calvert, G., Bullmore, E., Brammer, M., Campbell, R., Williams, S., McGuire, P., Woodruff, P., Iverson, S., & David, A. (1997). Activation of auditory cortex during silent lipreading. *Science, 276,* 593–596.

Carrell, T., Bradlow, A., Nicol, T., Koch, D., & Kraus, N. (1999). Interactive software for evaluating auditory discrimination. *Ear and Hearing, 20,* 175–176.

Cassandro, E., Mosca, F., Sequino, L., De Falco, F. A., & Campanella, G. (1986). Otoneurological findings in Friedreich's ataxia and other inherited neuropathies. *Audiology, 25,* 84–91.

Chisin, R., Perlman, M., & Sohmer, H. (1979). Cochlear and brain stem hearing loss following neonatal hyperbilirubinemia. *Annals of Otology, Rhinology and Laryngology, 88,* 352–357.

Davis, H., & Hirsh, S. (1979). A slow brainstem response for low-frequency audiometry. *Audiology, 18,* 445–461.

Deltenre, P., Mansbach, A. L., Bozet, C., Clercx, A., & Hecox, K. E. (1997). Auditory neuropathy: A report on three cases with early onsets and major neonatal illnesses. *Electroencephalography and Clinical Neurophysiology, 104,* 17–22.

Ferber-Viart Chantal, Duclaux, R., Dubreuil, C., Sevin, F., Collet, L., & Berthier, J. C. (1994). Otoacoustic emissions and brainstem auditory evoked potentials in children with neurological afflictions. *Brain & Development, 16,* 213–218.

Gatehouse, S. (1992). The time course and magnitude of perceptual acclimatization to frequency responses: Evidence from monaural fitting of hearing aids. *Journal of the Acoustical Society of America, 92,* 1258–1268.

Gorga, M. P., Stelmachowicz, P. G., Barlow, S. M., & Brookhouser, P. E. (1995). Case of recurrent, reversible, sudden sensorineural hearing loss in a child. *Journal of the American Academy of Audiology, 6,* 163–172.

Gravel, J., Kurtzberg, D., Stapells, D., Vaughan, H., & Wallace, I. (1989). Case studies. *Seminars in Hearing, 10,* 272–287.

Gravel, J., & Stapells, D. (1993). Behavioral, electrophysiologic, and otoacoustic measures from a child with auditory processing dysfunction: Case report. *Journal of the American Academy of Audiology, 4,* 412–419.

Gupta, A., Hans, R., & Anand, N. (1990). Auditory brainstem responses (ABR) in neonates with hyperbilirubinemia. *Indian Journal of Pediatrics, 57,* 705–711.

Hardin, A. (1995). From the syndrome of Charcot, Marie and Tooth to disorders of peripheral myelin proteins. *Brain, 118,* 809–818.

Harrison, R. (1988). An animal model of auditory neuropathy. *Ear and Hearing, 19,* 355–361.

Harrison, R., Stanton, S., Ibrahim, D., Nagasawa, A., & Mount, R. (1993). Neonatal cochlear hearing loss results in developmental abnormalities of the central auditory pathways. *Acta Otolaryngologica, 113,* 296–302.

Hienz, R., Stiles, P., & May, B. (1998). Effects of bilateral olivocochlear lesions on vowel formant discrimination in cats. *Hearing Research, 116,* 10–20.

Kalaydjieva, L., Hallmayer, J., Chandler, D., Savov, A., Nikolova, A., Angelicheva, D., King, R., Ishpekova, B., Honeyman, K., Calafell, F., Shmarov, A., Turnev, I., Hristova, A., Moskov, M., Stancheva, S., Petkova, I., Bittles, A., Georgieva, V., Middleton, L., & Thomas, P. (1996). Gene mapping in Gypsies identifies a novel demyelinating neuropathy on chromosome 8q24. *Nature Genetics, 14,* 214–217.

Koch, D., McGee, T., Bradlow, A., Kraus, N. (1999). An acoustic-phonetic approach toward understanding neural processes and speech perception. *Journal of the American Academy of Audiology, 10,* 304–318.

Kraus, N., Bradlow, A. R., Cheatham, M. A., Cunningham, J., King, C. D., Koch, D. B., Nicol, T. G., McGee, T. J., Stein, K. L., & Wright, B. A. (2000). Consequences of neural asynchrony: A case of auditory neuropathy. *Journal of the Association for Research in Otolaryngology, 1,* 33–45.

Kraus, N., & Disterhoft, J. (1982). Response plasticity of single neurons in rabbit auditory association cortex during tone-signalled learning. *Brain Research, 246,* 205–215.

Kraus, N., Koch, D., McGee, T., Nicol, T., & Cunningham, J. (1999). Speech-sound discrimination in school-age children: Psychophysical and neurophysiologic measures. *Journal of Speech, Hearing and Language Research, 41,* 1042–1060

Kraus, N., McGee, T., Carrell, T., King, C., Tremblay, K., & Nicol, T. (1995). Central auditory system plasticity associated with speech discrimination training. *Journal of Cognitive Neuroscience, 7,* 25–32.

Kraus, N., McGee, T., Carrell, T. D., Zecker, S. G., Nicol, T. G., & Koch, D. B. (1996). Auditory neurophysiologic responses and discrimination deficits in children with learning problems. *Science, 273,* 971–973.

Kraus, N., McGee, T., Ferre, J., Hoeppner, J., Carrell, T., Sharma, A., & Nicol, T. (1993). Mismatch negativity in the neurophysiologic/behavioral evaluation of auditory processing deficits: A case study. *Ear and Hearing, 14,* 223–234.

Kraus, N., McGee, T., & Koch, D. (1998). Speech-sound representation, perception and plasticity: A neurophysiologic perspective. *Audiology and Neuro-Otology, 3,* 168–182.

Kraus, N., Özdamar, Ö., Stein, L., & Reed, N. (1984). Absent auditory brain stem response: Peripheral hearing loss or brain stem dysfunction? *Laryngoscope, 94,* 400–406.

Lenhardt, M. (1981). Childhood central auditory processing disorder with brainstem evoked response verification. *Archives of Otolaryngology, 107,* 623–625.

Luce, P. A., & Pisoni, D. B. (1998). Recognizing spoken words: The neighborhood activation model. *Ear & Hearing, 19*(1), 1–36.

Lundberg, I., Frost, J., & Peterson, O. P. (1988). Effects of an extensive program for stimulating phonological awareness in preschool children. *Reading Research Quarterly, 23,* 263–284.

Merzenich, M., Grajski, K., Jenkins, W., Recanzone, G., & Peterson B. (1991). Functional cortical plasticity: Cortical network origins of representational changes. *Cold Spring Harbor Symposia on Quantitative Biology, 55,* 873–887.

Merzenich, M., Jenkins, W., Johnston, P., Schreiner, C., Miller, S., & Tallal, P. (1996). Temporal processing deficits of language-learning impaired children ameliorated by training. *Science, 271,* 77–81.

Naatanen, R., Schroger, E., Karakas, S., Tervaniemi, M., & Paavilainen, P. (1993). Development of neural representations for complex sound patterns in the human brain. *NeuroReport, 4,* 503–506.

Nakamura, H., Takada, S., Shimabuku, R., Matsuo, M., Matsuo, T., & Negishi, H. (1985). Auditory nerve and brainstem responses in newborns with hyperbilirubinemia. *Pediatrics, 75,* 705–708.

Nelson, K., Gilmore, R., & Massey, A. (1988). Acoustic nerve-conduction abnormalities in Guillain-Barre syndrome. *Neurology, 38,* 1263–1266.

Neville, H., Schmidt, A., & Kutas, M. (1983). Altered visual-evoked potentials in congenitally deaf adults. *Brain Research, 266,* 127–132.

Norton, S. (1993). Application of transient evoked otoacoustic emissions to pediatric populations. *Ear and Hearing, 14,* 64–73.

Picton, T. (1986). Abnormal brainstem auditory evoked potentials: A tentative classification. In R. Q. Cracco & I. Bodis-Wollner (Eds.), *Evoked potentials* (pp. 373–378). New York: AR Liss, Inc.

Picton, T. W., Stapells, D. R., & Campbell, K. B. (1981). Auditory evoked potentials from the human cochlea and brainstem. *Journal of Otolaryngology Supplement, 9,* 1–41.

Pisoni, D. B., Aslin, R. N., Perey, A. J., & Hennessy, B. L. (1982). Some effects of laboratory training on identification and discrimination of voicing contrasts in stop consonants. *Journal of Experimental Psychology, 8,* 297–314.

Prieve, B. A., Gorga, M. P., & Neely, S. T. (1991). Otoacoustic emissions in an adult with severe hearing loss. *Journal of Speech and Hearing Research, 34,* 379–385.

Reale, R., Brugge, J., & Chan, J. (1987). Maps of auditory cortex in cats reared after unilateral cochlear ablation in the neonatal period. *Developmental Brain Research, 34,* 281–290.

Recanzone, G., Schreiner, C., & Merzenich, M. (1993). Plasticity in the frequency representation of primary auditory cortex following discrimination training in adult owl monkeys. *Journal of Neuroscience, 13,* 87–104.

Robertson, D., & Irvine, D. (1989). Plasticity of frequency organization in auditory cortex of guinea pigs with partial unilateral deafness. *Journal of Comparative Neurology, 282,* 456–471.

Sams, M., Aulanko, R., Hamalainen, M., Hari, R., Lounasmaa, O., Lu, S. T., & Simola, J. (1991). Seeing speech: Visual information from lip movements modifies activity in the human auditory cortex. *Neuroscience Letters, 127,* 141–145.

Satya-Murti, S., Wolpaw, J. R., Cacace, A. T., & Schaffer, C. A. (1983). Late auditory evoked potentials can occur without brainstem potentials. *Electroencephalography and Clinical Neurophysiology, 56,* 304–308.

Sawada, M. (1979). Electrocochleography of ears with mumps deafness. *Archives of Otolaryngology, 105,* 475–478.

Schrott, A., Stephan, K., & Speondlin, H. (1989). Hearing with selective inner hair cell loss. *Hearing Research, 40,* 213–219.

Shankweiler, D., Crain, S., Katz, L., Fowler, A. E., Liberman, A. M., Brady, S. A., Thorton, R., Lundquist, E., Dreyer, L., Fletcher, J. M., Stuebing, K. K., Shaywitz, S. E., & Shaywitz, B. A. (1995). Cognitive profiles of reading-disabled children: Comparison of language skills in phonology, morphology, and syntax. *Psychological Science, 6,* 149–156.

Shapiro, S. M. (1994). Brainstem auditory evoked potentials in an experimental model of bilirubin neurotoxicity. *Clinical Pediatrics, 33,* 460–467.

Silver, S., Kapitulnik, J., & Sohmer, H. (1995). Contribution of asphyxia to the induction of hearing impairment in jaundiced Gunn rats. *Pediatrics, 95,* 579–583.

Sininger, Y. S., Hood, L. J., Starr, A., Berlin, C. I., & Picton, T. W. (1995). Auditory loss due to auditory neuropathy. *Audiology Today, 7,* 10–13.

Sininger, Y., Trautwein, P., Shallop, J., Fabry, L., & Starr, A. (1999). Electrical activation of the auditory nerve in patients with auditory neuropathy. *Assoc Res Otolaryngol Abstr, 22,* 170.

Starr, A., McPherson, D., Patterson, J., Luxford, W., Shannon, R., Sininger, Y., Tonokawa, L., & Waring, M. (1991). Absence of both auditory evoked potentials and auditory percepts dependent on time cues. *Brain, 114,* 1157–1180.

Starr, A., Picton, T. W., Sininger, Y., Hood, L. J., & Berlin, C. I. (1996). Auditory neuropathy. *Brain, 119,* 741–753.

Starr, A., Sininger, Y., Winter, M., Derebery, M. J., Oba, S., & Michalewski, H. J. (1998). Transient deafness due to temperature-sensitive auditory neuropathy. *Ear and Hearing, 19,* 169–179.

Stein, L., Tremblay, K., Pasternak, J., Banerjee, S., Lindemann, K., & Kraus, N. (1996). Brainstem abnormalities in neonates with normal otoacoustic emissions. *Seminars in Hearing, 17,* 197–213.

Tallal, P., Miller, S. L., Bedi, G., Byma, G., Wang, X., Nagarajan, S. S., Schreiner, C., Jenkins, W. M., & Merzenich, M. M. (1996). Language comprehension in language-learning impaired children improved with acoustically modified speech. *Science, 271,* 81–84.

Trautwein, P. G., Sininger, Y. S., & Nelson, R. (2000). Cochlear implantation of auditory neuropathy. *Journal of American Academy of Audiology, 11,* 309–315.

Tremblay, K., Kraus, N., & McGee, T. (1998). The time-course of auditory perceptual learning: Neurophysiological changes during speech-sound training. *Neuroreport, 9,* 3557–3560.

Tremblay, K., Kraus, N., Carrell, T., & McGee, T. (1997). Central auditory system plasticity: Generalization to novel stimuli following listening training. *Journal of the Acoustical Society of America, 102,* 3762–3773.

Vohr, B., White, K., & Maxon Johnson, M. (1993). Factors affecting the interpretation of transient evoked otoacoustic emission results in neonatal screening. *Seminars in Hearing, 14,* 57–72.

Weinberger, N. M., Hopkins, W., & Diamond, D. M. (1984). Physiological plasticity of single neurons in auditory cortex of the cat during acquisition of the pupillary conditioned response: I. Primary field (A1). *Behavioral Neuroscience, 98,* 171–188.

Worthington, D., & Peters, J. (1980). Quantifiable hearing and no ABR: Paradox or error? *Ear and Hearing, 5,* 281–285.

Patients With Auditory Neuropathy: Who Are They and What Can They Hear?

Yvonne Sininger and Sandy Oba

The disorder known as auditory neuropathy (Starr, Picton, Sininger, Hood, & Berlin, 1996) is not new but has recently become more clearly defined and understood. Until recently, the vast majority of hearing disorders that did not involve the conductive mechanism were felt to originate in the cochlea, usually due to dysfunction or loss of cochlear hair cells. This was true even though the literature was filled with case studies discussing what we would now call auditory neuropathy (AN; Kraus, Ozdamar, Stein, & Reed, 1984; Satya-Murti, Cacace, & Hanson, 1980; Spoendlin, 1974; Worthington & Peters, 1980). Some current estimates of incidence indicate that approximately 10% of the children seen with severe-to-profound deafness may have a neural rather than a hair cell disorder (Kraus et al., 1984; Rance et al., 1999).

A typical person with AN has the following profile: elevated thresholds on pure-tone audiogram by air and bone conduction, very poor speech discrimination for degree of loss, no acoustic reflex in any configuration for any stimuli, no auditory brain-stem response (ABR) even with stimuli that are well above detection threshold, evidence of large cochlear microphonic in auditory brain-stem response recordings and present otoacoustic emissions to low-level stimuli. A great number of nontypical cases of AN also can be included in this categorization, and it is appropriate to discuss the criteria that must be met to assume a diagnosis of AN in a patient.

To be considered as having AN, a patient must have *all* of the following:

1. **Evidence of poor auditory function (hearing).** The patient must have difficulty hearing in at least some situations or for some stimuli regardless of pure-tone thresholds. The case presented by Dr. Kraus in Chapter 1 is an example where threshold sensitivity may be reasonably normal but speech perception in noise is dysfunctional.

2. **Evidence of poor auditory neural function.** At a minimum, the patient must have elevated or absent auditory brain-stem reflexes (i.e., either middle ear muscle reflex or olivocochlear reflex) and abnormality of the ABR. For example, a very mild case might show poor ABR morphology or abnormal peak latency for fast clicks. A more common and severe manifestation would be no clear ABR waveform to any click stimuli at any level. When an ABR does appear, the threshold of the response will be significantly poorer than the psychophysical threshold for the eliciting stimuli, and the waveform morphology, peak amplitudes, or latencies will be abnormal.

3. **Evidence of normal hair cell function.** Most patients with AN demonstrate the presence of otoacoustic emissions (OAE), but a small percentage do not. A cochlear microphonic is also evidence of normal hair cell function and can be substituted for a normal OAE in the diagnosis of AN. One or the other must be seen to make the diagnosis of AN. It should be noted, however, that OAEs are evidence only of outer hair cell functioning; cochlear microphonics are generated by both inner and outer hair cells. Thus, there is presently no clear way to determine the functional status of the inner hair cell as distinct from the outer hair cells with these tests.

The purpose of this chapter is to describe in detail the patients with auditory neuropathy and their audiologic findings as summarized from our experience with a sample of this population. Results on other auditory functions will be discussed by Zeng et al. in Chapter 8. With the support of the National Institute of Deafness and Other Communicative Disorders, we have been studying patients with and characterizing the symptoms of this disorder for the last 5 years. Results of that work include a database containing details of 59 well-defined patients. Those data have allowed us to understand the heterogeneity as well as the common features of auditory neuropathy patients and their symptoms. Additional information on the physiologic and medical status of these patients can be found in Chapter 3 by Starr. A clear understanding of the range of findings will lead to a better understanding of the nature of the underlying physiology of this disorder and perhaps guide clinicians in determining appropriate intervention strategies. Findings on individual tests are provided here. A summary of information on the incidence of auditory neuropathy is provided, followed by case studies to illustrate how symptoms present in individuals.

PATIENTS WITH AUDITORY NEUROPATHY

Demographics

The mean age of onset of auditory neuropathy symptoms in our group of patients is 9 years. As shown in Figure 2–1, the range of onset is from birth to at least 60 years of age, with the largest group showing onset before 2 years of age. Seventy-five percent of the patients in our database were below 10 years of age when symptoms were first seen. There is an approximately equal distribution of male (55%) and female (45%) patients with auditory neuropathy.

Medical History

Only 27% of the patients with AN have no associated medical conditions or family history. Of the 25 patients with onset of symptoms before age 2, 80% had either family or neonatal risk factors. Table 2–1 shows a

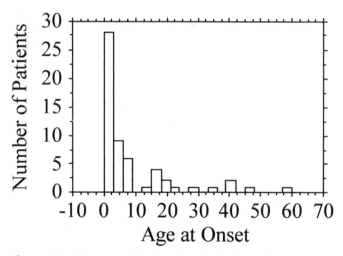

Figure 2–1. Histogram showing the distribution of age at onset from a database of 59 patients with auditory neuropathy.

Table 2–1. Patients with onset of auditory neuropathy before age 2 years, grouped by family history and other neonatal risk factors.

Risk Factors	Family or Genetic History		Total
	Yes	No	
Hyperbillirubinemia	2	1	3
Prematurity	1	1	2
Multiple risk factors	0	7	7
No other risk factors	8	5	13
Total	**11**	**14**	**25**

breakdown of neonatal risk factors and family and genetic history in the patients with early onset AN. Forty-eight percent of the infants (12 out of 25) have both family predisposition and neonatal risk factors indicating the possibility of a combination or interaction of effects. A genetic predisposition to hyperbillirubin toxemia might explain why some children with mild hyperbillirubinemia may later be found to have AN.

Our database indicated that 46% of AN patients had a family history of hearing disorder or a genetic basis for AN. Of 59 AN patients in our database, those with identified syndromes include 8 with hereditary sensory-motor neuropathy (Charcot-Marie-Tooth, Type I or II), 4 with Freidreich's ataxia, 1 with Stevens-Johnson syndrome, and 1 with Ehlers-Danlos syndrome. Four patients were reported with meningitis or other infectious disease. Reported complications or other conditions reported in the 59 patients with AN include seizures in 4 (7%); high fever in 2 (3%); and severe vision disorder, stroke, and torticollis in 1 each (2%).

AUDIOGRAMS

Degree and Configuration

Patients with auditory neuropathy present with all degrees of hearing loss from slight to profound. Figure 2–2 is a histogram of the pure-tone average hearing levels of our patients. The majority of our patients (82%) had symmetric losses; however, 14% had bilateral asymmetric losses, and about 4% were unilateral. Distribution of audiogram configuration is shown in Figure 2–3. Overall, 43% of patients show a flat audiometric shape, and 28% have a reverse sloping loss with higher thresholds for low-frequency stimuli than for high frequencies.

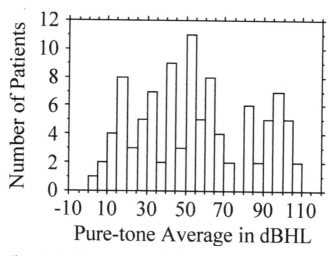

Figure 2–2. Histogram showing distribution of pure-tone average (PTA) hearing loss in dB HL from a database of 59 patients with auditory neuropathy.

Slope

The reverse slope of the audiogram in patients with AN can be quite dramatic as shown on the top of Figure 2–4. This configuration is further evidence that the underlying etiology of the hearing loss in AN is neural rather than cochlear, at least in patients with this dramatic reverse-slope configuration. The laws of basilar membrane mechanics, even passive mechanics, do not provide a viable explanation for significant loss of low-frequency sensitivity in light of much better high-frequency hearing. Even if all low-frequency sensory elements (hair cells) were missing, the traveling wave of the basilar membrane would cause displacement and excitation of high-frequency elements during low-frequency stimulation, producing a much more uniform response threshold curve than that shown in Figure 2–4.

One explanation for loss of sensitivity that is more dramatic for low frequencies relates to theories of pitch perception in which two mechanisms are postulated (see Moore, 1982, for discussion). High-frequency stimuli, especially those above 1000 Hz where refractory period limitations prevent temporal firing patterns from matching each cycle of stimulation, are felt to be signaled by the place of excitation (specific neural elements stimulated). Low-frequency stimuli may be encoded by temporal firing patterns, however, based on evidence that the refractory period could allow the normal auditory nerve to fire on each phase (or nearly each phase) of a low-frequency pure-tone signal. As we have seen repeatedly

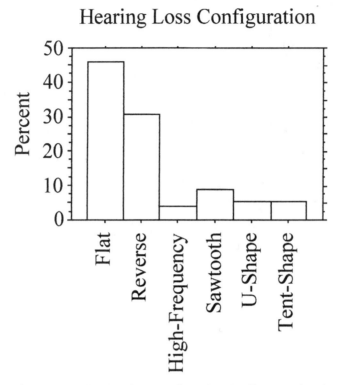

Figure 2–3. Hearing loss configuration (audiogram shape) distribution from a database of 59 patients with auditory neuropathy.

(see Zeng, Chapter 8), neural timing patterns are not synchronous with auditory stimuli in subjects with auditory neuropathy. Elevated low-frequency thresholds in patients with auditory neuropathy may be due to poor timing accuracy in the neural representation of low-frequency stimuli.

In contrast, normal or near-normal sensitivity for high-frequency stimuli reflects only detection of these stimuli, probably based on the mere presence of activity in a group of neurons, and may be unique to the task involved in the pure-tone audiogram. Normal detection thresholds, however, do not indicate normal signal processing. As an example of this, Figure 2–4 (at the bottom) shows the temporal modulation transfer function for the same subject whose audiogram is shown above (see Zeng, Chapter 8, for explanation of these procedures). Even though this patient has high-frequency detection thresholds that are within normal limits at 2 kHz and above, he has no detection of temporal modulations above

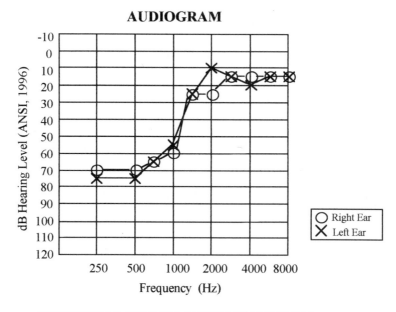

AUDIOGRAM

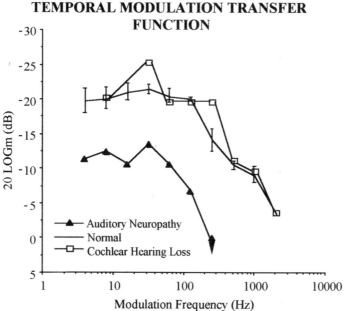

TEMPORAL MODULATION TRANSFER FUNCTION

Figure 2–4. Top: Audiogram from adult patient with AN demonstrating significant reduction in sensitivity for frequencies of 1000 Hz and below. **Bottom:** The temporal modulation transfer functions for the same patient shown in the audiogram above (triangles), for normal-hearing control subjects (solid line), and for one patient with low-frequency sensory loss (open squares). This patient's performance on the auditory perceptual task involving resolution of timing cues is significantly impaired for all frequencies, demonstrating that normal detection thresholds do not indicate normal auditory function in general.

100 Hz. In patients with AN, firing patterns for stimuli of all frequencies will be disordered and auditory tasks that are more complex than pure-tone detection, most notably speech perception, may be dysfunctional far beyond what is indicated by the audiogram.

Change in Hearing Over Time

Hearing loss progression in patients with AN has a different pattern than seen with sensory loss. As shown in Figure 2–5, 29% of patients with AN showed a significant amount (more than 10 dB pure-tone average) of fluc-

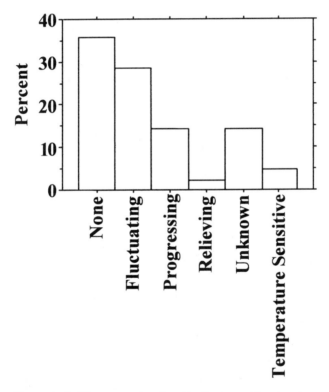

Figure 2–5. Histogram showing distribution of hearing loss progression over time from a database of 59 patients with auditory neuropathy. Fluctuating loss is defined as that in which there is more than 10 dB of change at three or more frequencies between tests but no predictable direction of change. Progressive cases are those that show similar change but in the direction of higher thresholds (poorer hearing) over time.

tuation in hearing level between tests. Fluctuating loss is distinguished from progressive loss (seen in 14% of patients with AN) because those with fluctuations do not show steadily increasing thresholds over time. An example of one case that shows particularly large fluctuations is shown in Figure 2–6. In fact, many patients with AN appear to have moment-to-moment fluctuations in hearing that can create the illusion of lack of cooperation or even malingering during the collection of pure-tone audiograms. Parents and teachers of children with AN repeatedly report that the children may have periods of "good hearing" and on other days appear deaf.

This inconsistency in neural representation of signals may be particularly disruptive to auditory learning and speech perception in the infant or young child with AN. In sensory loss, a weak, degraded signal, if consistent, can still form a basis for the learning of relationships between sound and meaning. If a given sound is represented to the brain in different ways and degrees from trial to trial, however, it is doubtful that appropriate associations can be made.

The most dramatic change in auditory status over time is demonstrated by patients who demonstrate what we call "temperature-sensitive" AN (Gorga, Stelmachowitz, Barlow, & Brookhouser, 1995; Starr et al., 1998). This disorder is quite rare, but we have seen three such patients, two of whom were siblings. These patients have hearing that is within normal limits when their core temperature is normal, but with fever of even a few degrees, they show significant loss of hearing sensitivity including severe-to-profound deafness. These patients have some of the standard findings of auditory neuropathy, including absent acoustic reflexes at all times, but when afebrile these patients have present, albeit abnormal, ABR and near-normal hearing and speech perception. Within minutes of fever striking, these patients' audiograms show severe-to-profound hearing loss, and the ABR disappears. Cochlear microphonics are clear and always present in these patients, as are OAEs.

In general, patients with AN can have any degree of hearing loss, and the day-to-day fluctuations in auditory capacity can be much more dramatic than are generally seen in patients with sensory loss.

SPEECH DISCRIMINATION

As previously noted (Sininger et al., 1995; Starr et al., 1996), patients with AN have dysfunction of speech perception that is out of proportion with their pure-tone loss. This is best illustrated by comparing speech discrimination scores in these patients to those expected by degree of hearing loss for patients with sensory loss (Yellin, Jerger, & Fifer, 1989). Figure 2–7 illustrates that when hearing loss pure-tone average exceeds about 30 dB,

AUDIOGRAM

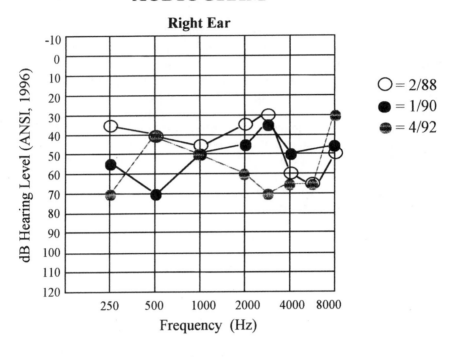

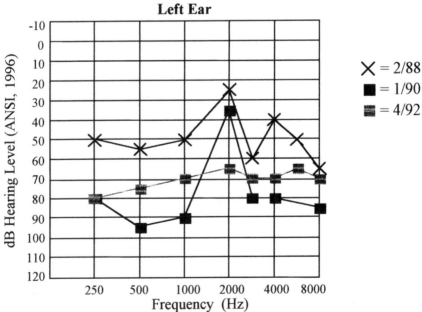

Figure 2–6. Demonstration of fluctuating hearing loss in one subject with auditory neuropathy.

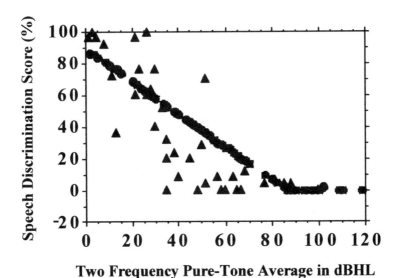

Figure 2–7. Circles indicate lower limit of expected speech discrimination scores in patients with sensory loss for average hearing loss level (on abscissa) predicted from Yellin et al. (1989). Triangles are actual scores on speech discrimination tests by average hearing level from patients with auditory neuropathy. Data from many subjects who were too young or who could not participate in a standard speech discrimination task are not shown.

the speech discrimination scores of AN patients from our sample (measured on standard CID W-22 lists) fall significantly below the level expected by Yellin et al. These data may be giving an optimistic look at speech discrimination in these patients because it could be measured on standard lists in less than half of our subjects overall and in only 10 of the 36 subjects under the age of 15.

These expected scores were originally developed to determine which patients might be suspect for an acoustic neuroma. Patients with AN, in fact, have many symptoms in common with those having acoustic neuroma, including poor speech discrimination, abnormal ABR, elevated or absent acoustic reflexes and, occasionally, present otoacoustic emissions. However, the vast majority of patients with tumors have unilateral disease, whereas most patients with auditory neuropathy have primarily bilateral involvement and are generally younger than those with tumors. Referral to neurology is always indicated to determine type and site of lesion whenever neural involvement is suspected.

ACOUSTIC REFLEX

Most patients with AN have no brain-stem auditory reflexes including acoustic (middle ear muscle) and olivocochlear reflex (for details on the latter, see Hood and Berlin, Chapter 10). In 44 of our patients in whom acoustic reflexes were measured, 93.5% showed absent reflexes and 6.5% (three cases) showed present or elevated reflexes.

OTOACOUSTIC EMISSIONS AND COCHLEAR MICROPHONIC

We described a case of AN a decade ago (Starr et al., 1991) without the benefit of OAEs. At that time, the diagnosis of retrocochlear dysfunction was based on the mismatch between the ABR and the audiogram (moderate loss on audiogram and no ABR), as well as the presence of a cochlear microphonic. Perhaps the most important factor in the recent increase in the number of diagnosed cases of AN is the advent of OAE testing in many clinical facilities. Such testing has revealed more patients with hearing loss and normal cochlear (outer hair cell) function than was previously appreciated.

In our sample, 80% of the patients with AN have a clear OAE. Only 9% have never shown an OAE during our evaluations, and in 11% the OAE disappeared over time. The amplitude distribution of transient-evoked otoacoustic emissions (TEOAEs) from our patients who show a response is given in Figure 2–8. In patients with AN, OAEs are strong but may not be abnormally large when the considering that our patient group is predominately children who typically display the largest amplitude OAEs (Norton & Widen, 1990).

Others have reported that patients with AN may have but later lose OAEs over time (Deltenre et al., 1999). The reason for loss of OAEs over time is unclear. Figure 2–9 shows that, for patients in our database, loss of OAEs happens most often in the young (mean age = 4.7 years), but the mean ages for those patient who still have or never have had OAEs is 16 and 18 years, respectively. Clouding the issue is the fact that when older AN patients present with absent otoacoustic emissions, it is possible that emissions may have been present at some time before our baseline testing. This can complicate the diagnosis of AN. The presence of a clear cochlear microphonic can supplant the presence of OAEs for meeting criterion three (evidence of normal hair cell function). In our database, all patients who were evaluated had a cochlear microphonic present and also had one or both of these signs (i.e., present OAE or cochlear microphonic). For a

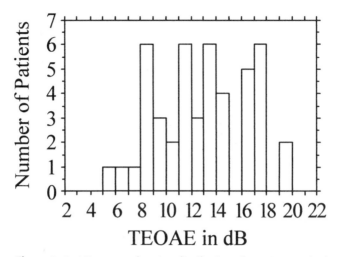

Figure 2–8. Histogram showing distribution of transient-evoked otoacoustic emission (TEOAE) amplitude from patients with auditory neuropathy.

more detailed discussion of cochlear microphonic and OAE see Starr, Chapter 3.[1]

Although we have observed loss of emissions over time in the older siblings of two sets of sibling pairs with AN, our data show that patients who lose their emissions have the same distribution of genetic (about one in three) and nongenetic (two in three) etiology as those who continue to exhibit emissions (see Chapter 9 on genetics). In addition, patients who lose their emissions over time are no more likely to have peripheral neuropathy than those with emissions. The reason for loss of emissions over time in patients with AN remains unclear.

[1] It is important that the cochlear microphonic be determined appropriately. The cochlear microphonic (CM) is seen as a large consistent series of peaks that occur early in the ABR recording and change polarity with the stimulus. The CM can be seen in a click-evoked ABR recording with a high-level stimulus (80 dB nHL). One average with a positive polarity click should be plotted on top of a recording with a negative polarity click. The CM will appear as mirror-image peaks that can last up to 5 or 6 ms in duration. The CM is only recorded from electrodes near the ear (ear lobe or mastoid). The cochlear microphonic will not be present at stimulus levels below about 60 dB nHL. It can be distinguished from a stimulus artifact by using an insert transducer. A cochlear microphonic will occur after the tubing-induced delay (usually about 0.6 ms) and, when tubing is clamped, the CM will disappear and stimulus artifact will be unaffected. The CM can be distinguished from wave I of the ABR because the polarity of the CM changes with stimulus polarity, which wave I does not, and because the latency of the CM does not change with stimulus level.

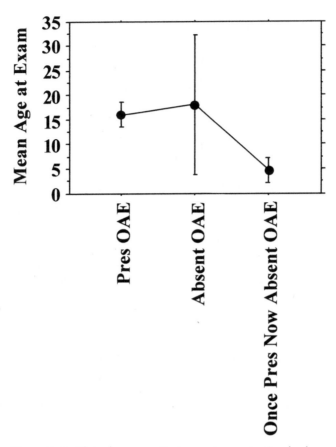

Figure 2–9. Plot of mean patient age at examination broken down by status of otoacoustic emissions (OAEs). Significantly lower age of subjects who have lost emissions indicates that emissions may disappear early in life for those subjects who lose them.

An important question regarding management of patients with AN is whether the use of hearing aids to help with the loss of sensitivity will cause acoustic trauma and possibly contribute to the loss of OAEs. Table 2–2 provides data on this question. More than half of the patients whose OAEs are still intact have used hearing aids, indicating that hearing aid use does not automatically cause a loss of OAEs. In fact, we have seen individual patients who came to us using high-gain amplification before the diagnosis of AN was made. In these few patients, OAEs may have been weak or absent following prolonged hearing aid use, but the

Table 2–2. Breakdown of otoacoustic emission (OAE) status by hearing aid use status.

Hearing Aid Status	OAE Present		OAE Absent		OAE Once Present Now Absent		All Patients	
	#	%	#	%	#	%	#	%
User	5	16	4	80	3	50	12	30
Past user	12	39	1	20	3	50	15	37
Never used	14	45	0	0	0	0	14	33
Total	31	100	5	100	6	100	42	100

Note: More than half of the patients with present OAEs have used or are using hearing aids. All of our patients with absent OAE have used amplification, however. Information on hearing aid use was not available on all patients.

OAE would return and be clear and robust following a week without amplification.

Table 2–2 also shows that all patients with absent or lost OAEs have used amplification at some time. Because of small numbers in these groups, it is not clear if this distribution is significantly different than expected, or if this is evidence that amplification may contribute to loss of OAEs. Further study is clearly warranted in this area, and the risk from use of amplification must be weighed against the benefits (if any) of amplification provided to the patient (see Cone-Wesson, Rance, and Sininger, Chapter 12, on rehabilitation).

AUDITORY BRAIN STEM RESPONSE RESULTS

Figure 2–10 shows a breakdown of the results of the ABR in our database. In this group, 70% of patients have a complete absence of any ABR waveform regardless of the level of the stimulus. Nineteen percent show wave V only, and in most of those, the peak is poorly defined, the latency is abnormal, and the amplitude is small. In 6% of our patients, we see an ABR that is abnormal but includes at least two of the traditional peaks, usually waves III and V. Again, the waveform morphology, including peak latency and amplitude, is clearly abnormal in these patients, but an ABR can be identified.

An apparent relationship exists between the degree of severity of the ABR result and the degree of hearing loss as shown in Figure 2–11. Those patients with absent ABR show the poorest pure-tone average thresholds and those with several peaks in the waveform (called abnormal ABR) have

Auditory Brain Stem Response Results

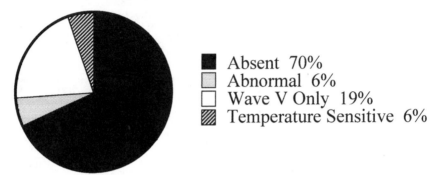

- ■ Absent 70%
- ▨ Abnormal 6%
- □ Wave V Only 19%
- ▨ Temperature Sensitive 6%

Figure 2–10. Pie chart of auditory brain stem response (ABR) results from a database of 59 patients with auditory neuropathy. Abnormal ABRs are characterized as having two or more peaks but significantly elevated thresholds relative to pure-tone average, as well as abnormal peak amplitude and latency. Temperature sensitive ABRs are those that are present yet abnormal when the patient is afebrile but disappear when the patient is febrile.

the best thresholds. In all cases of AN, however, the threshold of the ABR is unrelated to the hearing threshold. It is clear that the ABR cannot be used to estimate hearing thresholds in a patient with AN. Normal hair cell function must be ruled out in any patient, an infant for example, in whom ABR would traditionally be used for determining hearing level.

CASE STUDY

The data presented previously are statistically descriptive in nature. A case study is used here to illustrate the principles noted previously. Diagnostic test information on this patient is illustrated in Figure 2–12. The patient described is a boy of 7.5 years. He is generally in good health. His history includes one episode of fever, at age 3.5 years, that lasted 5 days and was accompanied by oral herpes. He has had recurrent otitis media treated with tympanostomy and ventilation tubes. Speech development was reportedly normal before age 5, but after that time, response to sound was inconsistent and speech development was slowed. Hearing evaluation did not reveal a loss at age 6 but by age 7, a moderate-to-severe hearing loss was discovered (see the audiogram in Figure 2–12). At that time, tympanometry was normal, acoustic reflexes were absent, and otoacoustic emissions were present.

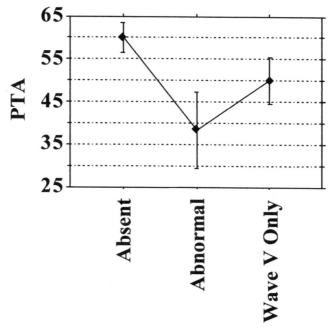

Figure 2–11. Graph shows average hearing level for patients with auditory neuropathy grouped by auditory brain stem response (ABR) abnormality. Abnormal ABRs have two or more peaks, wave V only has one peak, and absent ABRs have none. A loose association between degree of ABR abnormality and degree of hearing loss can be seen.

ABR testing revealed no response to 80 dB nHL stimuli, but evidence of a cochlear microphonic was seen in the recording. Magnetic resonance imaging of the brain and cranial nerves VII and VIII was normal, as was a neurologic examination.

Significant delays in expressive and receptive language have been documented, but articulation is generally age appropriate. Amplification and FM systems have been used sparingly with little success. This child relies heavily on speech-reading, supplemented with manual communication as necessary.

This child demonstrates a possible late-onset case of AN of unknown etiology. His audiogram shows the often-seen nonuniform configuration with peaks and valleys. We have noted significant fluctuations in his hearing over time. He is also typical in that he relies heavily on visual cues, including speech-reading, supplemented by signs, for receptive communication.

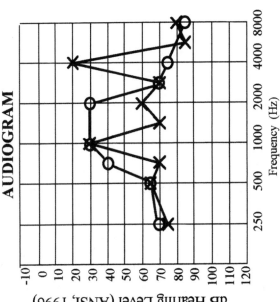

AUDIOGRAM

dB Hearing Level (ANSI, 1996)

Frequency (Hz)

Speech Awareness Threshold (SAT) -
Right Ear = 20 dBHL
Left Ear = 25 dBHL
Speech Discrimination -
Right Ear = 28%
Left Ear = 8%
Tympanometry = WNL
Acoustic Reflex Threshold = Absent

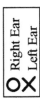

O Right Ear
X Left Ear

32

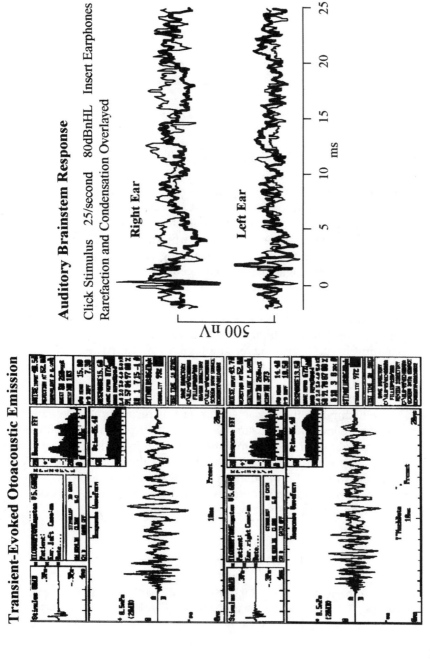

Figure 2–12. Audiogram, transient-evoked otoacoustic emissions and auditory brain stem responses from 7-year-old male patient with auditory neuropathy.

SUMMARY AND CONCLUSIONS

Patients with AN have all degrees of hearing loss, but many have losses in the severe-to-profound range. The pure-tone audiogram often has a flat or low-frequency emphasis configuration, but bizarre pure-tone loss configurations are common. The hearing loss of a patient with AN is more likely to fluctuate in a day-to-day or even minute-to-minute time frame than with sensory or conductive losses. Speech perception ability in patients with AN is dramatically poorer than predicted by the degree of hearing loss. The disorder can strike at any age, but most cases are congenital or occur in early childhood.

All patients with AN have absent or abnormal ABR and absent or severely elevated acoustic reflex thresholds. Some evidence of normal hair cell function must be seen to make an accurate diagnosis of AN. This evidence can be in the form of clear evidence of transient or distortion product OAEs or evidence of cochlear microphonic.

Auditory neuropathy is a heterogeneous disorder that has some common characteristics in auditory function but may have several etiologies and physiologic bases. For a complete characterization of medical and physiologic function in these same patients see Starr, Chapter 3; for details on auditory psychophysics evaluations, see Zeng et al., Chapter 8. Presently, only neural pathologies have been documented in these patients (Starr et al., 1996). The possibility of isolated inner hair cell dysfunction cannot be ruled out but has never been documented in any patient or in any known human temporal bone dissections. Consequently, until more accurate physiologic measures of inner hair cell function can be developed, it is appropriate to use the terminology of "auditory neuropathy" to define disorder that includes (a) hearing loss, (b) abnormal ABR (beginning with wave I) and brain stem reflexes, and (c) evidence of some current or previous normal hair cell function. Certainly, much more research is needed to distinguish the characteristics of this disorder and possible treatments. We believe that our sample of nearly 60 patients exhibiting this disorder should shed light on this subject for clinicians and researchers who see patients having AN, however. Whether this sample provides a good representation of this population remains to be seen. Coordination of clinical and research data and outcomes measures from centers worldwide would be helpful in further understanding this disorder.

REFERENCES

Deltenre, P., Mansbach, A. L., Bozet, C., Christiaens, F., Barthelemy, P., Paulissen, D., & Renglet, T. (1999). Auditory neuropathy with preserved cochlear microphonics and secondary loss of otoacoustic emissions. *Audiology (France), 38,* 187–195.

Gorga, M. P., Stelmachowicz, P. G., Barlow, S. M., & Brookhouser, P. E. (1995). Case of recurrent, reversible, sudden sensorineural hearing loss in a child. *Journal of the American Academy of Audiology, 6,* 163–172.

Kraus, N., Ozdamar, O., Stein, L., & Reed, N. (1984). Absent auditory brain stem response: Peripheral hearing loss or brain stem dysfunction? *Laryngoscope, 94,* 400–406.

Moore, B. C. J. (1982). *Introduction to the psychology of hearing.* London: Academic Press.

Norton, S. J., & Widen, J. E., (1990). Evoked otoacoustic emisssions in normal-hearing infants and children: Emerging data and issues. *Ear and Hearing, 11,* 121–127.

Rance, G., Beer, D. E., Cone-Wesson, B., Shepherd, R. K., Dowell, R. C., King, A. M., Rickards, F. W., & Clark, G. M. (1999). Clinical findings for a group of infants and young children with auditory neuroapthy. *Ear and Hearing, 20,* 238–252.

Satya-Murti, S., Cacace, A., & Hanson, P. (1980). Auditory dysfunction in Friedreich's ataxia: Result of spiral ganglion degeneration. *Neurology, 30,* 1047–1053.

Sininger, Y. S., Hood, L. J., Starr, A., Berlin, C. I., & Picton, T. W. (1995). Hearing loss due to auditory neuropathy. *Audiology Today, 7,* 10–13.

Spoendlin, H. (1974). Optic and cochleovestibular degenerations in hereditary ataxias. II. Temporal bone pathology in two cases of Friedreich's ataxia with vestibulo-cochlear disorders. *Brain, 97,* 41–48.

Starr, A., McPherson, D., Patterson, J., Don, M., Luxford, W. M., Shannon, R., Sininger, Y. S., Tonokawa, L. T., & Waring, M. (1991). Absence of both auditory evoked potentials and auditory percepts dependent on timing cues. *Brain, 114,* 1157–1180.

Starr, A., Picton, T. W., Sininger, Y., Hood, L. J., & Berlin, C. I. (1996). Auditory neuropathy. *Brain, 119,* 741–753.

Starr, A., Sininger, Y. S., Winter, M., Derebery, J., Oba, S., & Michalewski, H. (1998). Transient deafness due to temperature-sensitive auditory neuropathy. *Ear and Hearing, 19,* 169–179.

Worthington, D. W., & Peters, J. F. (1980). Quantifiable hearing and no ABR: Paradox or error? *Ear and Hearing, 1,* 281–285.

Yellin, M. W., Jerger, J., & Fifer, R. C. (1989). Norms for disproportionate loss in speech intelligibility. *Ear and Hearing, 10,* 231–234.

3

The Neurology
of Auditory Neuropathy

Arnold Starr

Auditory neuropathy is a term we first employed (Starr, Picton, Sininger, Hood, & Berlin, 1996) to characterize patients with a mild-to-moderate hearing disorder and a paradoxical absence or severe abnormality of the auditory brain stem response (ABR) beginning with wave I, the component generated by the distal auditory nerve. Tests of cochlear outer hair cell function including cochlear microphonics (CMs) and otoacoustic emissions (OAEs) were preserved. We interpreted the findings as consistent with a disorder of function of the auditory nerve. The disproportionate loss of auditory percepts dependent on temporal cues (Starr et al., 1991) suggested that there was an impairment of auditory neural synchrony. The presence of a concomitant peripheral neuropathy in many of the patients indicated that the auditory nerve dysfunction in these patients was due to a neuropathic disorder of the nerve, and thus the term "auditory neuropathy" seemed appropriate. We recognized that neural synchrony of the auditory nerve could also be affected if inner hair cells, synapses between inner hair cells and auditory nerve dendrites, or both were affected, but we had no ability to evaluate the likelihood of these alternative sites.

Peripheral and cranial neuropathies are a consequence of many different etiologies, such as infectious, degenerative, genetic, toxic-metabolic, immune, and so forth. The cranial nerves that are affected most frequently by neuropathic disorders are the optic, trigeminal, and facial nerves. In contrast, neuropathies of the auditory nerve are not typically recognized, the notable exception being a compression neuropathy of the auditory nerve accompanying acoustic neuromas.

This chapter reviews the neurology and physiology of approximately 70 patients with auditory neuropathy whom audiologists and otologists,

37

both locally and from around the country, referred to us. The results have helped establish that auditory neuropathies, as with other neuropathies, have diverse etiologies and varying expression of abnormal function. The data presented here are from the same group of patients described by Sininger and Oba in Chapter 2 of this volume.

CLINICAL FEATURES

Auditory neuropathy is typically bilateral (96%) and shows no gender preference: 46% of our sample are female patients, and 54% male patients. There are several factors that can be used to classify auditory neuropathies into distinct groupings. These include age of onset, the presence of a peripheral neuropathy, and physiologic measures of cochlear receptor and auditory nerve activities.

Etiology

Auditory neuropathies can be subdivided as to etiology (see Table 3–1) into hereditary (in approximately 40% of the subjects), a mix of etiologies

Table 3–1. Diagnoses of 70 patients with auditory neuropathy.

Hereditary (Total = 30)	
With peripheral neuropathy	**18**
Hereditary sensory motor neuropathy	(9)
Olivopontocerebellar	(1)
Freidreich's ataxia	(3)
Spinocerebellar degeneration	(2)
Leukodystrophy	(1)
Unknown	(2)
Without peripheral neuropathy	**12**
Others (Total = 15)	
Immune	1
Postinfectious	2
Hyperbilirubinemia	5
Premature	7
Idiopathic (Total = 25)	
Associated Diagnoses	
Ehrlers Danlos	1
Gonad dysgenesis	1
Seizures	4
Stevens Johnson	1

in 20% including toxic-metabolic (anoxia, hyperbilirubinemia), immuno-logic (drug reaction, demyelination), and infectious (postviral). No etiol-ogy (idiopathic) could be defined in almost 40% of affected individuals.

Auditory Neuropathy With Peripheral Neuropathy

The presence of a peripheral neuropathy was identified in 18 (27%) of the subjects with auditory neuropathy. The criteria used for diagnosing pe-ripheral neuropathy included one or more of the following: (a) clinical findings of absent ankle jerks or loss or abnormal reduction of vibration sense in the feet, (b) abnormal nerve conduction studies, and (c) abnormal sural nerve biopsy.

None of the children examined under the age of 5 years had clinical evidence of a peripheral neuropathy, therefore nerve conduction studies were not performed. There were two children between the ages of 5 and 10 years who had clinical and nerve conduction evidence of a peripheral neuropathy. In contrast, a peripheral neuropathy was defined in approxi-mately 80% of the subjects over 15 years of age. Thus, the association of auditory neuropathy and peripheral neuropathy is a common feature in adult but not young patients. In adults, the timing of the symptoms of peripheral and auditory neuropathy varied. In some, the disorder of pe-ripheral nerves occurred first, but in others hearing loss preceded symp-toms of weakness or sensory loss.

Thus, auditory neuropathies can occur in isolation or in association with a peripheral neuropathy. Assignment to these categories can change with maturation. For instance, the initial neurologic examination of two brothers with auditory neuropathy was normal. Two years later, the elder brother developed clinical signs of a peripheral neuropathy with abnor-mal nerve conduction studies. Regular examinations will help determine if young children with only hearing loss of the auditory neuropathy type will subsequently develop generalized peripheral neuropathy.

Table 3–1 details the diagnoses of the 18 patients with both periph-eral and auditory neuropathies. Hereditary sensory-motor neuropathy (HSMN), also known as Charcot-Marie-Tooth disease, affected nine indi-viduals from three families. The association of HSMN and hearing impair-ment had been noted frequently in the past (Harding, 1995), but tests to distinguish neuropathic from receptor loss were not available. The pheno-typic expression of HSMN is associated with several different genetic dis-orders (see Rogers, Chapter 9, this volume). We identified that in one HSMN family of Roma extraction in Slovenia, the mode of inheritance was recessive, and the genetic defect was localized to 8q24 (Butinar et al., 1999). The disorder is present in several other Roma families in Bulgaria (Kalaydjieva et al., 1996) with deafness and peripheral neuropathy. The clinical picture in the affected individuals with 8q24 deficit is of motor and sensory disabilities of the limbs appearing before age 20, with a hearing loss developing only later. There was also evidence of bilateral vestibular nerve involvement presumed to be due to the same neuropathic processes. The vestibular disorder was asymptomatic, probably due to the bilateral nature of the impairments and to the confinement of the patients to a wheelchair because of leg weakness. Testing of optic nerves was normal. Nerve conduction studies (three affected family members) and sural nerve biopsy (one affected family member) in this kindred were compatible, with a mixed axonal and demyelinating neuropathy that was rapidly progressive, affecting both motor and sensory nerves. We would expect that a similar type of pathology would characterize the auditory and vestibular nerves of affected family members.

In a second of our families with deafness and HSMN, the inheritance was dominant, whereas in the third family, the inheritance was recessive. The family with dominant inheritance had both a peripheral sensory motor neuropathy as well as an autonomic neuropathy. A sural nerve biopsy from one of the members of this family showed axonal loss with evidence of secondary demyelination and remyelination.

There were three individuals with a clinical diagnosis of Freidreich's ataxia (one with sporadic incidence, and two siblings of this individual) reflecting the association between deafness and Freidreich's reported by others (Spoendlin, 1974). Sural nerve biopsy from one of the siblings showed axonal neuropathy. There were two individuals in the database with spinocerebellar degeneration. Sural nerve biopsy (Figure 3–1) from one of these patients also showed an axonal disorder with demyelination and remyelination of the remaining axons. A normal sural nerve is shown for comparison in the figure. There was one individual with olivopontocerebellar atrophy (also known as multiple system atrophy); one with an unspecified type of leukodystrophy, a myelin disorder of central nerve fibers; and one individual with the clinical and laboratory features of an inflammatory demyelinating peripheral neuropathy.

The variety of diagnoses above represents the diversity of etiologies we have encountered that affect both peripheral and auditory nerves. The list of etiologies is more extensive when we include reports in the literature of deafness due to auditory nerve involvement with Guillain-Barre syndrome, an immune disorder (Ropper & Chiappa, 1986; Schiff, Cracco, & Cracco, 1985), multiple sclerosis (Marangos, 1996), and diabetes mellitus (Parving et al., 1990).

The neuropathologies of the few sural nerve biopsies from our patients with auditory neuropathy have shown pathology of axons, myelin, or a combination of the two (see Chapter 5 for additional details). We assume the auditory nerve would be similarly affected in these individuals. We need additional experience to define whether the type of neuropathology relates to the hearing impairments or to measures of cochlear or auditory nerve function.

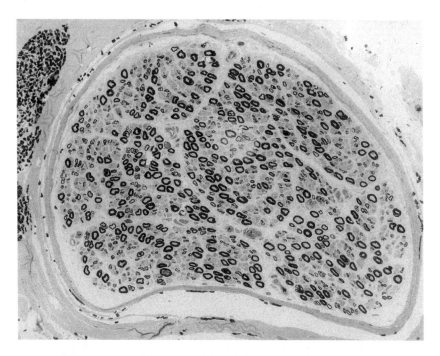

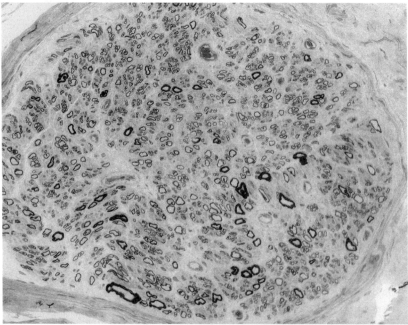

Figure 3–1. Cross section of a normal sural nerve biopsy (top) and a sural nerve from an auditory neuropathy subject (below) with a concomitant peripheral neuropathy. The magnification is ×280. Note the loss of large myelinated fibers in the subject with auditory neuropathy and the thinning of myelin in many of the remaining large fibers.

41

Auditory Neuropathy Without Peripheral Neuropathy

Approximately two thirds of the patients with auditory neuropathy have no evidence of a concomitant peripheral neuropathy. There are several possible reasons for this. First, the patients without a peripheral neuropathy were typically children in whom the expression of the peripheral nerve disorder may lag that of the auditory nerve. Second, the neuropathy may be selective for just the auditory nerve as can be found in other cranial neuropathies. Third, there may be alternative mechanisms (e.g., synaptic disorder or inner hair cell disorder) accounting for auditory nerve dysfunction.

We had the opportunity to study three subjects with an isolated auditory neuropathy whose clinical and laboratory measures suggested that disordered neural transmission (a conduction block of auditory nerve fibers) was the primary problem in these subjects (Gorga et al., 1995; Starr et al., 1998). When afebrile, the children had hearing within the normal range but abnormal ABRs beginning with wave I. They would become profoundly deaf with febrile episodes. Treatment with acetaminophen that dropped body temperature to normal was accompanied by a return of their hearing. Although the children appeared to have almost normal hearing when afebrile, other test results were compatible with auditory neuropathy. Wave I of the ABR was absent, whereas wave V was delayed in latency and reduced in amplitude. OAEs were normal; CMs and a summating potential were preserved; middle ear muscle reflexes were absent. During the febrile events, OAEs remained normal, ABRs were lost, and both speech comprehension and pure-tone thresholds were profoundly impaired. A striking temperature-dependent loss of neural function is also seen in demyelinating disorders of the nervous system, such as multiple sclerosis. We proposed that these children have a demyelinating disorder confined to their auditory nerves.

The site of involvement of the auditory nerve in patients with auditory neuropathy is almost always in the distal segment because wave I of the ABR, which is generated within the temporal bone, is usually absent. An involvement of the proximal portion of the 8th nerve was identified in one subject with auditory neuropathy who had a preserved wave I and absence of wave II, the latter generated by the 8th nerve adjacent to the brain stem. This subject has a myelin disorder (leukodystrophy) affecting the oligodendroglia, the source of myelin for the proximal portions of the 8th nerve (see Moore and Linthicum, Chapter 6).

The possibility that alternative sites in the auditory periphery may be involved in dysfunction of the auditory nerve is supported by the finding that there were some instances in which the absence of the ABR was sensitive to changes in stimulus rate. In three subjects, no ABR components were found at the standard stimulus rate (circa 20/s), but a clear wave V was evident at slower rates of stimulation (see Starr, Picton, and Kim's Chapter 5 on neural mechanisms in this volume). The mechanisms by which stimulus rate in subjects with normal hearing affects ABR amplitudes and latencies have been attributed to synaptic processes. In these individuals, a 20/s rate has minimal effects, but the loss of the ABR in patients with auditory neuropathy when using this conservative stimulus rate is striking. A disorder of the synapse between inner hair cells and 8th nerve dendrites could account for such rate sensitivity in these patients.

Relationships Among Auditory Nerve, Brain Stem, and Receptor Functions in Auditory Neuropathy

Acoustic Brain Stem Reflexes

Middle ear muscle reflex contractions in response to acoustic signals were absent in all but four of the patients with auditory neuropathy. The muscle reflex loss cannot be due to a disorder of the efferent components of the system (facial nerve and stapedius muscle) because nonacoustic middle ear muscle reflexes to tactile facial stimulation were present when examined in two patients with auditory neuropathy (Gorga et al., 1995; Starr et al., 1998). The disorder of acoustic middle ear responses must lie in the afferent limb of the reflex comprising the auditory nerve and cochlear nucleus connections to the 7th cranial nucleus. The brain stem reflexes governing crossed suppression of OAEs via olivocochlear bundle activation were evaluated in 13 of our subjects and found to be absent in all, findings similar to results of Hood and Berlin, Chapter 10 in this volume.

The loss of these brain stem reflexes is puzzling because there are no other signs of brain stem impairment, and hearing thresholds can be almost normal. Acoustic middle ear reflexes normally are engaged when sounds are intense and evoke high rates of discharge in the auditory nerve and afferent pathway to activate motor neurons of the stapedius muscle. The disorder of auditory nerve function (Starr et al., 1991; Zeng, Oba, Garde, Sininger, & Starr, 1999; Zeng et al., Chapter 8 in this volume) that we believe to be the hallmark of auditory neuropathy may provide the basis for the loss of acoustic brain stem reflexes. In auditory neuropathy, the auditory nerve may not achieve a sufficiently high rate of discharge to activate acoustic reflex contractions of middle ear muscles or the crossed olivocochlear reflex (see Starr, Picton, and Kim, Chapter 5 in this volume for further details).

Hair Cell Measures: Cochlear Microphonics

The surface recordings (Cz-ipsilateral mastoid) we employed for the ABR also revealed CM components that could be distinguished from artifacts by attention to recording and stimulus techniques (Berlin et al., 1998; Starr et al., in press). Results from a control subject and a patient with auditory neuropathy are shown in Figure 3–2 in response to condensation and rarefaction clicks presented separately.

A plot of the amplitude of the maximum CM component in 33 subjects with auditory neuropathy and 13 control subjects as a function of age is shown in Figure 3–3. There was a significant inverse linear correlation between age and CM amplitude in normals ($p = .01$, $r = -.54$). The individual measures of CM amplitude for AN subjects also showed a correlation with age, but the amplitudes of many of the measures were abnormally elevated (> 2 SD above the age adjusted mean of healthy subjects). There were 13 subjects with auditory neuropathy (21 ears), all less than 10 years of age, who exhibited abnormally increased CM amplitudes. These individuals comprised 54% of subjects with auditory neuropathy in this age group. Clinical features (such as the presence of neonatal risk factors, peripheral neuropathy, and the presence of auditory neuropathy in other family members) also correlated with subject age and therefore did not distinguish subjects with the disorder who had normal and abnormally elevated CMs.

Hair Cell Measures: OAEs

OAEs were absent in approximately 30% of subjects with auditory neuropathy (see Sininger and Oba, Chapter 2 in this volume). In the 21 subjects for whom transient evoked OAEs (TEOAEs) were bilaterally present, there was a significant inverse linear relationship between response amplitude and subject age ($r = -.38$, $p < .01$, intercept at 14.7 dB). TEOAE amplitudes were significantly correlated between ears ($p < .01$; $r = .63$). The correlation between the amplitudes of TEOAEs and CMs from the same ear when TEOAEs were present ($n = 33$) was also significant ($r = .45$, $p < .01$).

Hair Cell Measures: Conclusions

There are several mechanisms that could affect an increase in CM amplitude in patients with auditory neuropathy. First, graded contractions of the middle ear muscles can selectively enhance transmission of certain tonal frequencies and effect a slight increase in CM (Pilz, Ostwald, Kreiter, & Schnitzler, 1997; Starr, 1969), but we consider this alternative unlikely. Second, in experimental animals, activation of the efferent olivocochlear bundle (OCB) can lead to a doubling of amplitude of the CM (Fex, 1962; Galambos, 1956). OCB activation causes hyperpolarization of outer hair cells with an accompanying increase in receptor potentials and a decrease in neural activity of the 8th nerve (Fex, 1959). Crossed suppression

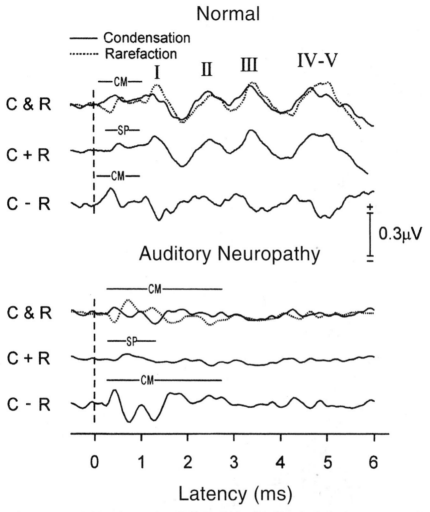

Figure 3–2. Auditory brain stem response from a healthy control subject (8 year old, top) and a subject with auditory neuropathy (5 year old, bottom) recorded from vertex to the mastoid ipsilateral to the acoustic stimulus are superimposed in the top traces (C & R) of each record to separately presented condensation (C) and rarefaction (R) click stimuli. Roman numerals (I through V identify neural components) and cochlear microphonics (CM) are identified by their phase reversal. Phase-reversed components are attenuated when the two averages are added (C + R) and enhanced when the averages are subtracted (C − R). A summating potential (SP) on the rising slope of wave I is marked in the C + R trace. Zero ("0") in the time base refers to the time of arrival of the sound stimulus at the eardrum. Note the presence of CM and SP in both subjects and the presence of neural components only in the healthy control.

Cochlear Microphonics

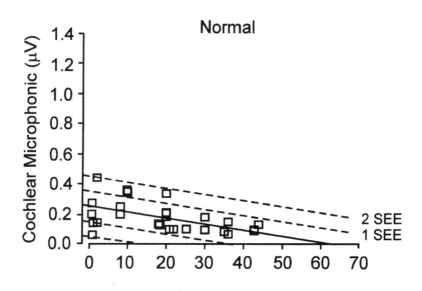

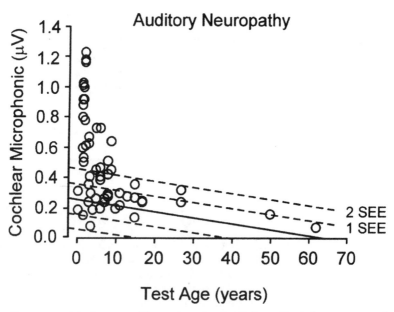

Test Age (years)

Figure 3–3. Maximum cochlear microphonic (CM) amplitude from 25 control ears (upper graph) and 57 auditory neuropathy ears (lower graph) as a function of subject age. In control subjects, there was a significant negative linear change of CM amplitude and age; 1 and 2 standard errors for control subjects are indicated. In subjects with auditory neuropathy, there was a clustering of abnormally elevated CM values for subjects less than 10 years of age.

of OAEs in auditory neuropathy is absent (Berlin et al., 1993), suggesting that OCB function is altered in this disorder. If the disorder of the OCB system took the form of tonic overactivity, CMs could be of large amplitude. Finally, pharmacologic agents, such as acetylsalicylic acid, can influence hair cell metabolism leading to an increase in CM amplitudes (Aran & De Sauvage, 1975). It may be that some subjects with auditory neuropathy harbor a metabolic disorder of hair cells leading to enhanced CMs and an accompanying impairment of afferent auditory nerve activity.

The loss of OAEs in a number of AN subjects may be evidence of outer hair cell dysfunction in some patients with this disorder. Numerous technical issues need clarification to be certain of the significance of the finding, however. Even with the above limitations, we are of the opinion that both the CM and TEOAE alterations found in subjects with auditory neuropathy, in this and in other studies (Deltenre et al., 1999; Rance et al., 1999), provide a strong presumption that cochlear dysfunction can be involved in this disorder. We are unable to distinguish whether the alterations of cochlear hair cell functions are a cause or a consequence of disordered auditory nerve activity in these patients. The relationship between neurons along a pathway is affected by the function of the pathway. Loss of neurons can lead to transsynaptic degeneration of neurons, whereas increased use of a pathway can lead to enhancement of neuronal synaptic structures. We can envision that disorders affecting the function of synapses between hair cells and auditory nerve, such as a neuropathy or an inner hair cell disease, would likely have profound influences on the structure and function of both elements.

Auditory Brain Stem Potentials

The presence of wave V, without a preceding wave I, was identified in the ABR from 12 (38%) of our 33 AN subjects. Seven of the subjects with ABRs were assessed bilaterally (4 subjects had a wave V from stimulating each ear; 3 had a wave V from stimulating only one of the ears). The mean amplitude of wave V when present (16 ears with auditory neuropathy) was 0.1 μV, significantly ($p < .01$) less than the mean amplitude of wave V in normal subjects (0.51 μV). Wave V latency in auditory neuropathy was delayed in 10 of the 16 recordings (6.0 ms to 8.5 ms).

The finding of a preserved wave V in a minority of subjects with the disorder is objective evidence that the disorder of auditory nerve synchrony varies. Auditory neuropathy is not a single entity but shows gradations of impairments affecting degree of hearing loss (Rance et al., 1999; Zeng et al., 1999), receptor functions (Starr et al., in press), and auditory pathway responses. These and other observations provide the bases to identify the varieties of hearing loss that comprise the condition we now label as "auditory neuropathy."

SUMMARY

Analyses of clinical features indicate that auditory neuropathies vary in several measures including age of onset, presence of peripheral neuropathy, etiology, and behavioral and physiologic measures of auditory function. These variations could represent the usual spectrum of a single disease. Alternatively, they may suggest that "auditory neuropathy" actually comprises several different disorders that vary as to both the site(s) of abnormality (dendrites or axons of the auditory nerve, outer and inner hair cells) and the pathophysiologic processes acting at those sites.

The disorder can to be progressive in a significant number of subjects as evidenced by loss of OAEs over time, a slight progression in the extent of hearing loss, or development of symptoms of peripheral neuropathy. We have not encountered subjects whose hearing loss or objective measures have improved substantially over time. Our knowledge of the natural history of the hearing disorder in subjects with auditory neuropathy is incomplete because we are in the early stages of following a substantial number of subjects. Our understanding of this disorder will grow as we have the opportunity to study, evaluate, and follow more patients.

Acknowledgments: Work described in this chapter was supported by the National Institute on Deafness and Other Communicative Disorders Grant No. DC02618.

REFERENCES

Aran, J.-M., & De Sauvage, R. C. (1975). Normal and pathological adaptation of compound VIII nerve responses in the guinea pig. *Acta Otolaryngologica, 79,* 259–265.

Berlin, C. I., Hood, L. J., Cecola, P., Jackson, D. F., & Szabo, P. (1993). Does Type I afferent neuron dysfunction reveal itself through lack of efferent suppression? *Hearing Research, 65,* 40–50.

Butinar, D., Zidar, J., Leonardis, L., Popovic, M., Kalaydjieva, L., Angelicheva, D., Sininger, Y., Keats, B., & Starr, A. (1999). Hereditary auditory, vestibular, motor, and sensory neuropathy in a Slovenian Roma (Gypsy) kindred. *Annals of Neurology, 46,* 36–44.

Deltenre, P., Mansbach, A. L., Bozet, C., Christiaens, F., Barthelemy, P., Paulissen, D., & Renglet, T. (1999). Auditory neuropathy with preserved cochlear microphonics and secondary loss of otoacoustic emissions. *Audiology, 38,* 187–195.

Fex, J. (1959). Augmentation of cochlear microphonic by stimulation of efferent fibers to the cochlear. *Acta Oto-Laryngology, 50,* 540–541.

Fex, J. (1962). Auditory activity in centrifugal and centripetal cochlear fibres in cat: A study of a feedback system. *Acta Physiologia (Stockholm) Supplement, 55,* 189.

Galambos, R. (1956). Suppression of auditory nerve activity by stimulation of efferent fibres to cochlea. *Journal of Neurophysiology, 19,* 424–437.

Gorga, M. P., Stelmachowicz, P. G., Barlow, S. M., & Brookhouser, P. E. (1995). Case of recurrent, reversible, sudden sensorineural hearing loss in a child. *Journal of the American Academy of Audiology, 6,* 163–172.

Harding, A. E. (1995). From the syndrome of Charcot, Marie and Tooth to disorders of peripheral myelin proteins. *Brain, 118,* 809–818.

Kalaydjieva, L., Hallmayer, J., Chandler, D., Savov, A., Nikolova, A., Angelicheva, D., King, R. H. H., Ishpekova, B., Honeyman, K., & Calafell, F. (1996). Gene mapping in Gypsies identifies a novel demyelinating neuropathy on chromosome 8q24. *Nature Genetics, 14,* 214–217.

Marangos, N. (1996). Hearing loss in multiple sclerosis: Localization of the auditory pathway lesion according to electrocochleographic findings. *Journal of Laryngology and Otology, 110,* 352–357.

Parving, A., Elberling, C., Balle, V., Parbo, J., Dejgaard, A., & Parving, H.-H. (1990). Hearing disorders in patients with insulin-dependent diabetes mellitus. *Audiology, 29,* 113–121.

Pilz, P. K., Ostwald, J., Kreiter, A., & Schnitzler, H. U. (1997). Effect of the middle ear reflex on sound transmission to the inner ear of rat. *Hearing Research, 105,* 171–182.

Rance, G., Beer, D. E., Cone-Wesson, B., Shepherd, R. K., Dowell, R. C., King, A. M., Rickards, F. W., & Clark, G. M. (1999). Clinical findings for a group of infants and young children with auditory neuropathy. *Ear and Hearing, 20,* 238–252.

Ropper, A. H., & Chiappa, K. H. (1986). Evoked potentials in Guillain-Barré syndrome. *Neurology, 36,* 587–590.

Schiff, J. A., Cracco, R. Q., & Cracco, J. B. (1985). Brainstem auditory evoked potentials in Guillain-Barré syndrome. *Neurology, 35,* 771–773.

Spoendlin, H. (1974). Optic and cochleovestibular degenerations in hereditary ataxias. II. Temporal bone pathology in two cases of Friedreich's ataxia with vestibulo-cochlear disorders. *Brain, 97,* 41–48.

Starr, A. (1969) Regulatory mechanisms of the auditory pathway. In S. Locke (Ed.), *Modern neurology* (pp. 101–114). Boston: Little, Brown and Co.

Starr, A., McPherson, D., Patterson, J., Don, M., Luxford, W. M., Shannon, R., Sininger, Y. S., Tonokawa, L. T., & Waring, M. (1991). Absence of both auditory evoked potentials and auditory percepts dependent on timing cues. *Brain, 114,* 1157–1180.

Starr, A., Picton, T. W., Sininger, Y., Hood, L. J., & Berlin, C. I. (1996). Auditory neuropathy. *Brain, 119,* 741–753.

Starr, A., Sininger, Y. S., Winter, M., Derebery, J., Oba, S., & Michalewski, H. (1998). Transient deafness due to temperature-sensitive auditory neuropathy. *Ear and Hearing, 19,* 169–179.

Starr, A., Sininger, Y., Nguyen, T., Michalewski, H., Oba, S., & Abdala, C. (in press). Cochlear receptor (microphonic and summating potentials, otoacoustic emissions) and auditory pathway (auditory brainstem potentials) activity in auditory neuropathy. *Ear and Hearing.*

Zeng, F. G., Oba, S., Garde, S., Sininger, Y., & Starr, A. (1999). Temporal and speech processing deficits in auditory neuropathy. *NeuroReport, 10,* 3429–3435.

Models of Auditory Neuropathy Based on Inner Hair Cell Damage

Robert V. Harrison

The term *auditory neuropathy* was originally used to describe hearing disorders in which there was found to be incongruency between various measures of auditory function, for example, an absent or abnormal auditory brain stem evoked response (ABR) that did not correspond to the patient's audiometric thresholds, or poorer speech discrimination scores than expected based on the patient's audiometric status. In addition, objective tests of cochlear function using otoacoustic emissions (OAEs; or, before their discovery, of cochlear microphonic [CM] recordings) showed many subjects to have better (outer) hair cell function than might be predicted from their psychophysical performance (Berlin, Hood, Cecola, Jackson, & Szabo, 1993; Deltenre, Mansbach, Bozet, Clercx, & Hecox, 1997; Starr et al., 1991; Stein et al., 1996; Worthington & Peters, 1980; for review, see Starr, Picton, Sininger, Hood, & Berlin, 1996).

The observations of relatively normal OAEs (or robust CM) in many of these patients indicates that damage to the outer hair cells is not the primary cause of auditory neuropathy. This, to many, was a surprising finding given the commonly held notion that the outer hair cells (OHCs) are particularly vulnerable and causally implicated in many types of sensorineural hearing loss (e.g., acoustic trauma, aminoglycoside ototoxicity, and presbyacusis). As demonstrated in the studies presented in this chapter however, it is the inner hair cell (IHC)/cochlear afferent system that appears to be much more fragile than the OHC to a variety of cochlear insults.

Another important observation in subjects with auditory neuropathy is that the ABR waveform is severely abnormal beginning at wave I, which suggests that the disorder arises from a cochlear pathology or the 8th nerve rather than some more central lesion (Starr et al., 1996). This narrows down the anatomic location of auditory neuropathy to somewhere along the auditory pathway between the outer hair cells and afferent neurons of the auditory nerve. It would be convenient if we could define the exact site of damage that results in auditory neuropathy; however that will be difficult given that auditory neuropathy, as presently defined, most likely has more than one etiology. In addition, damage to one part of the peripheral auditory system tends to result in secondary degenerative effects. For example, IHC loss is invariably followed by spiral ganglion cell degeneration and atrophy of second-order sensory neurons. In the animal models of auditory neuropathy presented here, the initial site of the functional damage is at the level of the IHC and its synapse with the primary afferent neuron. Our models certainly represent one subset of the condition in humans, arguably the most common etiology.

One of the intriguing features of auditory neuropathy is that (behavioral) audiometric thresholds (perhaps showing a mild-to-moderate sensorineural hearing loss) can be markedly better than ABR thresholds. This means that if there is cochlear damage, it is not extensive enough to prevent some relatively low-threshold cochlear afferent activity across a range of frequency locations. On the other hand, to reduce the number of synchronized neurons that contribute to the ABR, the deterioration has to be quite significant. We propose that such conditions could arise from scattered IHC loss, with minimal OHC damage.

Two types of animal model relating to auditory neuropathy are reported here. In the first model, subjects (chinchillas) have a chronic condition characterized by extensive but not total (i.e., scattered) inner hair cell degeneration and normal outer hair cells. Functionally, these animal subjects display many of the characteristics seen in patients with auditory neuropathy; they have normal OAEs (and CM), whereas ABR thresholds are significantly elevated. However, single-unit recordings from the auditory midbrain (inferior colliculus) show near-normal response thresholds. The scattered IHC damage in this model was produced by carboplatin (an antineoplastic agent). This does not reflect a naturally arising condition; however, we review evidence that similar scattered IHC loss can also arise from a mild, sustained cochlear hypoxia. We propose this latter mechanism as a likely cause of auditory neuropathy in humans.

Our second model explores the differential vulnerability of the IHC and OHC systems to hypoxia and, in separate experiments, to glutamate infusion into the cochlea. Results from these experiments strongly support the notion that chronic cochlear hypoxia, similar to that which might be experienced in some "high-birth-risk infants," can damage the IHC system independently of the outer hair cells. Much of the data presented here has been formally published elsewhere (Harrison 1998; Takeno, Harrison, Ibrahim, Wake, & Mount, 1994; Takeno, Harrison, Mount, Wake, & Harada, 1994; Takeno, Wake, Mount, & Harrison, 1998; Wake, Anderson, Takeno, Mount, & Harrison, 1996; Wake, Takeno, Ibrahim, & Harrison, 1993, 1994; Wake, Takeno, Mount, & Harrison, 1996).

MODELS

The first animal model of auditory neuropathy presented here is a chronic preparation in which scattered IHC loss is produced by treatment of chinchillas with the anticancer agent carboplatin. In this model, I describe the functional consequences of scattered IHC loss on IHC-mediated neural activity (as revealed by cochlear action potentials [CAP], ABR, or single-unit recording in the midbrain). In addition, OHC function is measured using OAE or CM recording.

The second animal model involves acute experiments that explore the differential effects of chronic cochlear hypoxia and glutamate instillation on IHC and OHC systems. In these experiments, the focus is on the independent monitoring of OHC function using OAE and of the IHC/primary afferent complex using ABR measures. In both experimental series, we have made histologic studies of the cochleas. The experimental methods are briefly described below; the reader can gain more details from the publications referenced.

Animal Model 1: Chronic Studies With Carboplatin

For carboplatin-induced IHC lesions, adult chinchillas (500–700 g) were treated with 400 mg/m^2 IV carboplatin (Paraplatin-AQ; Bristol Myers, Canada). All electrophysiologic recordings (ABR, CAP, CM) were made in the ketamine-anesthetized animals. ABRs were recorded using skin needle electrodes in a standard vertex to postaural configuration. Calibrated acoustic stimuli were short (1 ms rise/fall, 2 ms plateau) tone pips between 0.5 and 8 kHz. Evoked potentials were bandpass filtered (150 Hz–3 kHz) and amplified conventionally. After A–D conversion and artifact rejection, signals were averaged (Cambridge Electronic Design 1401).

For CAP and CM recordings, a silver ball electrode was surgically placed on the round window of the cochlea using a dorsal approach through the roof of the bulla. Stimuli used for CAP recordings were as those described above for the ABRs. For CM recording, no signal averaging was employed, and low-pass filters were removed to allow recording of the 8 kHz CM. For all the potentials, waveform amplitudes were measured over a range of stimulus intensities near to threshold allowing CAP and ABR threshold determinations; for CM, a "threshold" criterion of

10 mV was used. In carboplatin-treated animals, pretreatment ABR potentials were recorded followed by posttreatment ABR, CAP, and CM data collection from eight cochleas of five carboplatin-treated animals (see Takeno, Harrison, Ibrahim et al., 1994, for further details).

Transient evoked otoacoustic emissions (TEOAEs) were measured using the ILO88 (otodynamics) system to record from the ear canals of the lightly anaesthetized chinchillas. Stimuli used were clicks at a rate of 50 per sec, intensity 85 ± 3 dB SPL using the nonlinear mode (for more details, see Wake, Anderson et al., 1996).

Microelectrode studies in the auditory midbrain (inferior colliculus) were performed in the ketamine-anesthetized subject. Ketamine (15 mg/kg), xylazine (2.5 mg/kg), and atropine (0.004 mg/kg) supplemented as required during experiments. After a bilateral parietal craniotomy, occipital cortex was removed to expose the midbrain. A calibrated, closed-sound delivery system was used. All recordings were undertaken in a sound attenuated and electrically shielded room. Single unit recordings in response to pure-tone stimuli (70 ms duration and 10 ms rise and fall) were made in the inferior colliculus (central nucleus) using tungsten microelectrodes. For each neuron, the response area (to sound frequency and intensity; frequency threshold curve) was determined (for more technical details, see Harrison, Kakigi, Hirakawa, Harel, & Mount, 1996).

Animal Model 2: Acute Hypoxia Experiments

Chronic cochlear hypoxia was achieved by adding a 20 mL of dead space to the tidal volume of the respiratory tract of the tracheotomized animal. Subjects were maintained for 2 to 3 hours in this condition of mild hypoxia. Before and throughout this period, OAEs and ABRs were continuously recorded. TEOAE and ABR measures were made in a similar manner to that described above. Distortion product otoacoustic emissions (DPOAEs) were measured from the ear canal using the ILO92 system (Otodynamics, London). In general, equal-level primaries at 50 dB SPL with an f2/f1 ratio of 1:1.2 were used and the $2f_1$-f_2 emission was monitored. Periodically throughout the experiment, full ABR and DPOAE input–output functions were also measured to stimuli centered at 8 kHz.

Histologic Studies

Scanning electron microscopy of the cochlea was routinely done after all experiments. This involved systemic (aortic) perfusion followed by local cochlear perfusion of fixative (phosphate buffered 1% glutaraldehyde–4% formaldehyde), immediately postmortem. Cochleas were postfixed with 1% $0s0_4$ and dissected in 70% alcohol. After dissection, specimens were prepared using osmium-thiocarbohydrazide-osmium (OTO) procedures (Shirane & Harrison, 1987b) and critical point dried. Some cochlear specimens were also fixed, decalcified, embedded, and sectioned for light microscopy, using standard techniques.

All procedures involving animal subjects were performed within strict standards required by the University of Toronto Animal Care Committee under the guidelines set by the Canadian Council on Animal Care.

RESULTS AND DISCUSSION

Animal Model 1

Carboplatin-induced damage in the chinchilla cochlea is characterized by various degrees of IHC degeneration but with little damage to the OHC. The images of Figure 4–1 illustrate this differential damage to the IHC versus OHC. The upper four panels show scanning electron micrographs (SEMs) of the surface of the sensory epithelium from various cochlear positions. The lower panel is a light microscopic section through an area of the sensory epithelium showing (three) normal OHC, but no IHC (note the conspicuous gap in the area next to the inner pillar cell).

In the right-hand panels of Figure 4–2, cochleograms from four carboplatin-treated animals are shown. For each subject, the whole length of the cochlea has been assessed (using SEM) and the number of surviving IHC and OHC is plotted. The examples are arranged in order of increasing severity of damage. Importantly, note that while IHC damage can be extensive along the cochlear length, it is not total. There is a tendency for more damage toward the basal region of the cochlea (for more details see Takeno, Harrison, Mount et al., 1994). It is also important to note that when the IHC degenerate in these animals, so do the spiral ganglion cells (primary cochlear afferents) that were connected to them. This retrocochlear degeneration subsequent to IHC loss has been well documented in other studies, including the seminal work of Spoendlin (1975). A close correlation between IHC loss and cochlear afferent degeneration was recently confirmed in our animal model (Takeno et al., 1998). In addition to cochlear afferent degeneration, further pathologic changes ensue in second- and third-order neurons along the auditory pathway (e.g., Jean-Baptiste & Morest 1975; Morest & Bohne 1983; Powell & Erulkar, 1962). Thus, although the entity of auditory neuropathy might originate with a cochlear lesion, consequent central effects will certainly develop.

Auditory function in these animals shows many of the characteristics associated with auditory neuropathy in human subjects, as we will describe below.

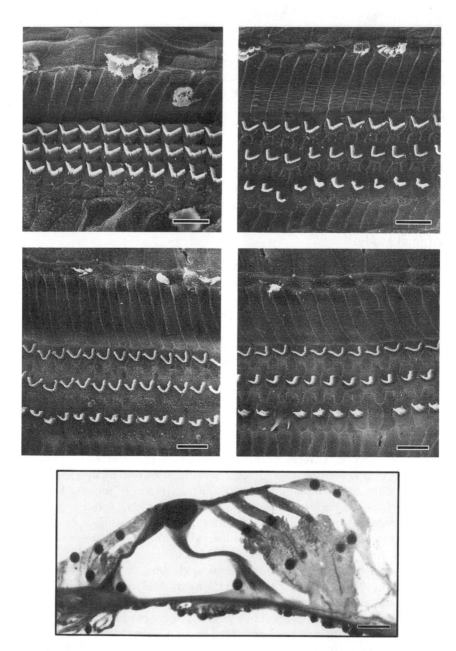

Figure 4–1. The effects of carboplatin treatment on inner and outer hair cells of the chinchilla cochlea. The four upper panels show scanning electron micrographs of the cochlear sensory epithelium taken from various cochlear positions and illustrate the general finding of degeneration of inner hair cells, whereas outer hair cells appear normal. Scale bar = 10μm. The lower panel shows a light microscopic view through a region having normal outer hair cells (three rows clearly seen) but no inner hair cells (note the clear gap adjacent to inner pillar cell). Scale bar = 10μm.

Measures of Neural Function

When evoked potential thresholds (CAP or ABR) to frequency-specific stimuli (tone pips) are measured in these animals, the loss of IHC (and cochlear afferents) is revealed by elevated thresholds. In Figure 4–2, the left-hand panels indicate the elevations in ABR thresholds (to frequency-specific stimuli) resulting from the carboplatin-induced cochlear lesions shown in the adjacent cochleograms. Note the general correlation between ABR signal changes and the degree of IHC loss. For example, in the subject depicted in the two uppermost panels, a 50% loss of IHC resulted in 20–30 dB ABR threshold change. More extensive hair cell loss, such as in the animal shown in the two lower panels, results in a 50–70 dB ABR threshold shift. We believe that these evoked potential thresholds are elevated not because the underlying neuronal units have elevated response thresholds, but because the number of activated neural elements is so reduced that the remotely recorded compound action potential signal is reduced in amplitude.

This notion has been confirmed by recording from single units of the inferior colliculus (IC) in these models. Figure 4–3 shows the results from two such experiments. Data from normal control subjects are illustrated in the uppermost graph, which shows the typical close correlation between ABR (wave V equivalent) threshold (dotted line) and the single unit minimum thresholds of IC neurons. This relationship appears to break down in animals with reduced neuronal density as shown in the two examples. The right-hand panels show the ABR threshold versus single-unit data corresponding to the cochleograms of hair cell damage indicated in the left panels. In both examples, at frequencies above 1 kHz (corresponding to cochlear regions with extensive IHC loss), ABR thresholds are significantly elevated, by as much as 30–50 dB, in comparison with single-unit neuronal thresholds. On the other hand, ABR thresholds to low-frequency stimulation (500 Hz) correspond well to the minimum thresholds of neurons, corresponding to apical areas of the cochlea having relatively good IHC survival. Note, importantly, that the individual IC neurons have relatively normal response thresholds. This situation is directly analogous to the observation in many patients with auditory neuropathy that ABR thresholds do not correlate with audiometric (behavioral) thresholds. In the case of our animal model, we have not tested behavioral thresholds, but rather infer from the single unit data that low-threshold information is reaching the central auditory system.

We also infer from our data that although some low-threshold information is being passed by the surviving IHC and their central connections, the amount of information (here, for humans, read speech information) that can be passed is diminished according to the reduced number of information channels. Thus, a cochlea with only 10–20% of IHCs surviving

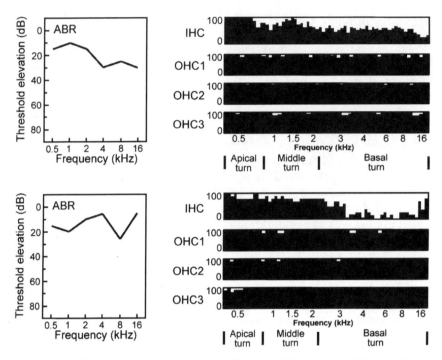

Figure 4–2. Effects of selective inner hair cell loss on ABR thresholds. The right-hand cochleograms show the pattern of cochlear hair cell deterioration in four chinchillas after treatment with carboplatin. The data are vertically arranged according to the degree of inner hair cell damage. Note that there is little outer hair cell loss in any of these subjects. The ABR audiograms for these subjects are shown in the left-hand panels and indicate ABR threshold elevations relative to the pretreatment values.

can only transfer a limited amount of (speech) information. In humans this information loss would be particularly noticeable in the reduction of speech information transmitted. How much actual information loss there is depends on how much redundancy there is in the system. It may be that the channel capacity can be significantly reduced before spectral and temporal information in speech starts to be degraded. At a qualitative level, however, I argue that complex auditory tasks including speech signal recognition could be significantly impaired and incongruent with audiometric threshold data.

Otoacoustic Emission Measurements

In some of the earliest reports of auditory neuropathy, it was observed that the cochlear microphonic was often prominent (i.e., more than would

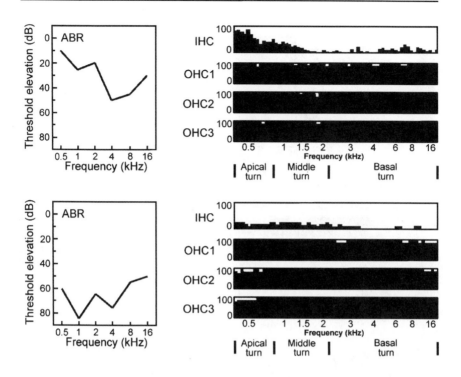

be expected given the degree of hearing loss). Later studies in which OAE testing was done in patients revealed that OAE amplitudes were much greater than expected based on the general degree of hearing dysfunction and, in some cases, were found to be abnormally large. In our animal model, the survival of OHC after carboplatin treatment results, perhaps not surprisingly, is demonstrated in the preservation of OAEs. In Figure 4–4, for two subjects, example transient evoked OAEs are shown before (left panels) and after (right panels) cochlear lesions in which the hair cell degeneration is as indicated by the cochleogram (center panels). It is evident that in these two examples, the OAEs are not only preserved but are increased in amplitude as a result of the IHC loss. This observation has been noted in some patients with auditory neuropathy (Berlin, personal communication, March 1998).

Animal Model 2

It is clear that in most human subjects with auditory neuropathy the cause is not carboplatin drug treatment. A "natural" mechanism for producing IHC damage is long-term cochlear hypoxia. Our research group has previously reported the effects of long-term hypoxia on the cochlea in exper-

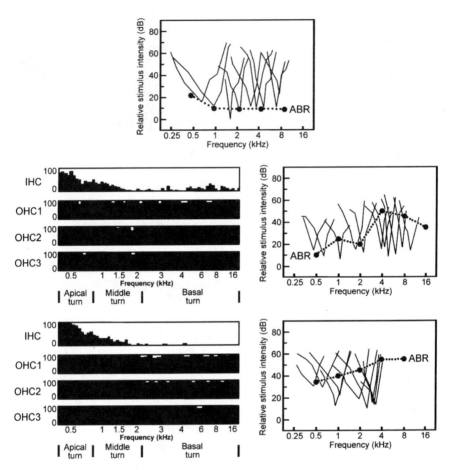

Figure 4–3. Comparison of frequency-specific ABR and response thresholds of single units in the inferior colliculus (IC). The top panel shows a sample of single-unit tuning curves (frequency threshold curves) from a normal control chinchilla compared with ABR thresholds to tone pip stimuli (dotted line joining filled symbols). The two sets of data below are from carboplatin-treated animals. The pattern of hair cell damage is indicated by the cochleograms (left), and the single-unit tuning curves versus ABR thresholds are shown in the right-hand panels. Note that after extensive (but subtotal) inner hair cell degeneration, there is poor correlation between ABR threshold and IC neuronal thresholds.

imental animals. For example, after a period of about 3 hours of mild hypoxia, IHC swelling and other damage was demonstrated in cochlear regions where OHC appeared normal (Shirane & Harrison, 1987a, 1987b). Figure 4–5 shows two example SEMs from the surface of the cochlear

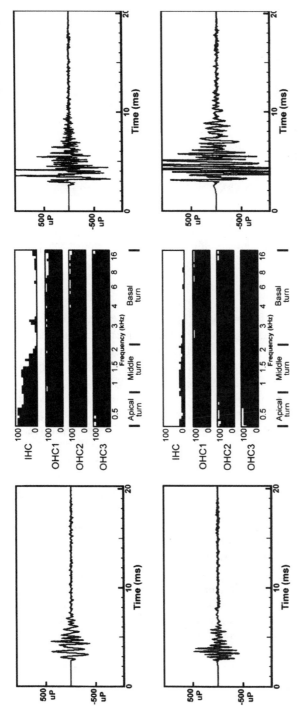

Figure 4–4. Examples of two subjects in which transient evoked otoacoustic emissions were measured, using identical stimulus parameters, before (left-hand panels) and after (right-hand panels) carboplatin treatment in the chinchilla. The cochleograms (center panels) show the pattern of cochlear hair cell degeneration in the two subjects; there is relatively little degeneration to the outer hair cell population.

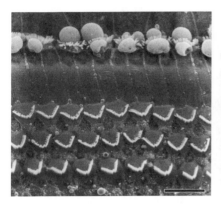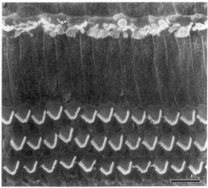

Figure 4–5. The effects of chronic hypoxia on cochlear hair cells. The two example SEM photomicrographs show the inner hair cell blebbing (cytoplasmic extrusion secondary to membrane disruption) resulting from a 3-hour period of mild hypoxia. Scale bar = 10μm.

sensory epithelium after prolonged mild hypoxia, demonstrating an apparently greater change to the IHC (cytoplasmic extrusion, disruption of stereocilia) compared with the OHC. Other histologic studies have also described the vulnerability of the IHC–afferent synapse in hypoxic conditions (Billet, Thorne, & Gavin, 1989; Bohne, 1976).

Effects of chronic cochlear hypoxia are explored in our second type of animal model of auditory neuropathy. OHC function using OAEs, and IHC–cochlear afferent activity using ABR, have been continuously monitored during periods of long-term cochlear hypoxia. Figure 4–6 shows a typical result. The upper plots show threshold changes to ABR potentials (filled circle symbols; scale on left ordinates) compared to DPOAE amplitude (left panel; open squares) and to TEOAE amplitudes (right panel; open triangles) during and after a 180-min hypoxic period (horizontal bar). In this example, after approximately 2 hours of hypoxia, the neural (ABR) potentials started to deteriorate, while the OHC function (as reflected in the OAEs) remained relatively unchanged. After normal conditions are restored (end of bar symbol), the differential dysfunction persisted to the end of the 250-min recording session. After this experimental period, cochlear examination using SEM demonstrated the pathologic conditions similar to those shown in Figure 4–5 (i.e., evidence of damage to the IHC region, but no evidence of pathologic change to the OHC). Such mild, chronic hypoxia is proposed as a candidate for causing auditory neuropathy, especially in patients with history of high-risk birth or in certain disorders that affect energy metabolism.

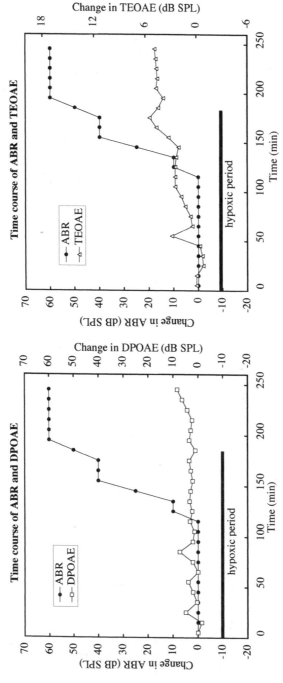

Figure 4–6. The differential changes to neural (ABR) thresholds and to otoacoustic emission signals during and after a 3-hour period of mild cochlear hypoxia. The left-hand plot shows DPOAE amplitudes (open square symbols; scale on left) together with ABR thresholds (filled symbols; scale on left). The right-hand plot shows TEOAE amplitudes with (the same) ABR threshold data. The period of hypoxia is indicated by the horizontal bar on each plot.

Etiology of Auditory Neuropathy

The reported cases of auditory neuropathy vary in terms of suggested etiology. It has definitely been associated with a number of hereditary disorders including Charcot-Marie-Tooth disease (e.g., Berlin et al., 1993), Friedreich's ataxia (Taylor, McMenamin, Andermann, & Walters, 1982), and various other hereditary motor and sensory neuropathies (Starr et al., 1996). Other etiologies implicated are kernicterus (Kaga, Kitazumi, & Kadama, 1979) and perhaps cisplatin drug treatment (Hansen, 1992). Other reports have associated auditory neuropathy with high-risk-birth infants (see Chapter 2 by Sininger and Oba). Clearly, an abnormally prolonged parturition could result in a period of cochlear hypoxia. We have also observed auditory neuropathy symptoms in a child having had a fetal maternal blood transfusion and also in case of shaken baby syndrome (Hospital for Sick Children, Toronto, unpublished data), both of which implicate cochlear hypoxic events.

Our animal models strongly suggest that many of the symptoms of auditory neuropathy are consistent with a pattern of cochlear hair cell damage in which OHC are relatively normal in function, but in which there is extensive, scattered but subtotal IHC loss. The research described here suggests that similar changes can result from chronic, mild hypoxia and that this represents one possible "natural" etiology for auditory neuropathy.

Acknowledgments: The work described has been carried out in the Auditory Science Laboratory by a number of collaborators to whom I am indebted. These include Mr. Richard Mount, Dr. Makoto Shirane, Dr. Mark Wake, Dr. Sacchio Takeno, and Dr. Shoichi Sawada. The studies reported here were supported by Medical Research Council (Canada) and the Masonic Foundation of Ontario.

REFERENCES

Berlin, C. I., Hood, L. J., Cecola, P., Jackson, D. F., & Szabo, P. (1993). Does type I afferent neuron dysfunction reveal itself through lack of efferent suppression? *Hearing Research, 65,* 40–50.

Billett, T. E., Thorne, P. R., & Gavin, J. B. (1989). The nature and progression of injury in the organ of Corti during ischemia. *Hearing Research, 41,* 189–198.

Bohne, B. A. (1976). Mechanisms of noise damage in the inner ear. In D. Henderson, R. P. Hamernik, D. S. Dosanjh, & J. H. Mills (Eds.), *Effects of noise on hearing* (pp. 41–68), New York: Raven.

Deltenre, P., Mansbach, A. L., Bozet, C., Clercx, A., & Hecox, K. E. (1997). Auditory neuropathy: A report on three cases with early onsets and major neonatal illnesses. *Electroencephalography and Clinical Neurophysiology, 104,* 17–22.

Hansen, S. W. (1992). Late-effects after treatment for germ-cell cancer with cisplatin, vinblastine, and bleomycin. *Danish Medical Bulletin, 39,* 391–399.

Harrison, R. V. (1998). An animal model of auditory neuropathy. *Ear & Hearing, 19,* 355–361.

Harrison, R. V., Kakigi, A., Hirakawa, H., Harel, N., & Mount R. J. (1996). Tonotopic mapping in auditory cortex of the chinchilla. *Hearing Research, 100,* 157–163.

Jean-Baptiste, J., & Morest, D. K. (1975). Transneuronal changes of synaptic endings and nuclear chromatin in the trapezoid body following cochlear ablation in cats. *Journal of Comparative Neurology, 162,* 111–133.

Kaga, K., Kitazumi, E., & Kadama, K. (1979). Auditory brain stem responses of kernicterus infants. *International Journal of Pediatric Otorhinolaryngology, 1,* 255–264.

Morest, D. K., & Bohne, B. A. (1983). Noise induced degeneration in the brain and representation of inner and outer hair cells. *Hearing Research, 9,* 145–151.

Powell, T. S., & Erulkar, S. D. (1962). Transneuronal cell degeneration in the auditory relay nuclei of the cat. *Journal of Anatomy, 96,* 249–268.

Shirane, M., & Harrison, R. V. (1987a). The effects of hypoxia on sensory cells of the cochlea. *Scanning Microscopy, 1,* 1175–1183.

Shirane, M., & Harrison, R. V. (1987b). The effects of deferoxamine mesylate and hypoxia on the cochlea. *Acta Otolaryngologica, 104,* 99–107.

Spoendlin, H. (1975). Retrograde degeneration of the cochlear nerve. *Acta Otolaryngologica, 79,* 266–275.

Starr, A., McPherson, D., Patterson, J., Don, M., Luxford, W., Shannon, R., Sininger, Y., Tonokawa, L., & Waring, M. (1991). Absence of both auditory evoked potentials and auditory percepts dependent on timing cues. *Brain, 114,* 1157–1180.

Starr, A., Picton, T. W., Sininger, Y., Hood, L. J., & Berlin, C. I. (1996). Auditory neuropathy. *Brain, 119,* 741–753.

Stein, L., Tremblay, K., Pasternak, J., Bannerjee, S., Lindemann, K., & Kraus, N. (1996). Brainstem abnormalites in neonates with normal otoacoustic emissions. *Seminars in Hearing, 17,* 197–213

Takeno, S., Harrison, R. V., Ibrahim, D., Wake, M., & Mount, R. J. (1994). Cochlear function after selective inner hair cell degeneration induced by carboplatin. *Hearing Research, 75,* 93–102.

Takeno, S., Harrison, R. V., Mount, R. J., Wake, M., & Harada, Y. (1994). Induction of selective inner hair cell damage by carboplatin. *Scanning Microscopy, 8,* 97–106.

Takeno, S., Wake, M., Mount, R. J., & Harrison, R. V. (1998). Degeneration of spiral ganglion cells in the chinchilla after inner hair cell loss induced by carboplatin. *Audiology and Neurotology, 3,* 281–290.

Taylor, M. J., McMenamin, J. B., Andermann, E., & Watters, G. V. (1982). Electrophysiological investigation of the auditory system in Friedrich's ataxia. *Canadian Journal of Neurological Science, 9,* 131–135.

Wake, M., Takeno, S., Ibrahim, D., & Harrison, R. V. (1993). Carboplatin ototoxicity: An animal model. *Journal of Otology and Laryngology, 107,* 585.

Wake, M., Takeno, S., Ibrahim, D., & Harrison, R. V. (1994). Selective inner hair cell ototoxicity induced by carboplatin. *Laryngoscope, 104,* 488-493.

Wake, M., Anderson, J., Takeno, S., Mount, R. J., & Harrison, R. V. (1996). Oto-acoustic emission amplification after inner hair cell loss. *Acta Otolaryngologica, 116,* 374–381.

Wake, M., Takeno, S., Mount, R. J., & Harrison, R. V. (1996). Recording from the inferior colliculus following cochlear inner hair cell damage. *Acta Otolaryngologica, 116,* 714–720.

Worthington, D. W., & Peters, J. (1980). Quantifiable hearing and no ABR: Paradox or error? *Ear and Hearing, 1,* 281–285.

Pathophysiology
of Auditory Neuropathy

Arnold Starr, Terence W. Picton, and Ronald Kim

Hearing loss can result from (a) decreased sound conduction into the cochlea, (b) reduced transduction of sound by the inner hair cells in the cochlea, (c) abnormal transmission of impulses by the fibers of the auditory nerve, or (d) disordered processing in the central auditory pathways. Physiologic measurements make it possible to distinguish among the latter three types of hearing loss, which are otherwise categorized together as "sensorineural." Auditory evoked potentials (Picton, 1990; Starr & Don, 1988) assess the function of the auditory nerve and central nervous system. Otoacoustic emissions (Probst, Lonsbury-Martin, & Martin, 1991) and cochlear microphonics (Berlin et al., 1998; Starr et al., in press) can demonstrate the function of the hair cells.

We used these physiologic measurements to identify a group of 10 patients (Starr, Picton, Sininger, Hood, & Berlin, 1996) with hearing impairment, normal otoacoustic emissions (OAEs), cochlear microphonics (CM), or a combination thereof and an absence or severe abnormality of the auditory brain stem response (ABR) beginning with wave I. Seven of the 10 patients had an accompanying neuropathy of the peripheral nervous system. We proposed that the findings were consistent with a neuropathic disorder of the auditory nerve in the presence of normal cochlear function, and we used the designation of "auditory neuropathy" for these patients (Starr et al., 1996). We suggested that the hearing loss reflected an involvement of the auditory nerve either as part of a generalized peripheral neuropathy or as an isolated auditory nerve disorder.

Individuals with a peripheral neuropathy of acute or subacute onset have symptoms of sensory loss, unusual sensations (paresthesia), uncomfortable sensations (dysesthesia), and weakness and muscle atrophy if motor nerve fibers are also involved. These symptoms are muted if the neuropathy is of gradual onset and slowly progressive, however. With sensory neuropathies, the neurologic examination reveals elevated thresholds for sensation, rapid adaptation to a stimulus, and altered perception of the specific quality of sensation. The deep tendon reflexes are often absent or hypoactive, reflecting the involvement of the large sensory nerve fibers originating from muscle receptors in the tested muscle.

Individuals with auditory neuropathy have symptoms that might be analogous to those accompanying a peripheral neuropathy. There is sensory loss reflected by elevated thresholds and decreased hearing affecting speech comprehension, particularly when there is a noisy background. Paraesthesiae such as tinnitus are rare, however, and loud sounds generally are not experienced as uncomfortable. Details of the subjective auditory experiences of two adults with AN are included in the preface to this book.

The pathophysiology leading to a combination of impaired auditory nerve function (abnormal ABRs) in the presence of preserved cochlear receptor function (normal OAEs or CMs) can theoretically occur in several ways. The organ of Corti consists of an afferent division (inner hair cells and afferent nerve fibers) that transduces sounds to neural activity and an efferent division (outer hair cells and efferent nerve fibers) that facilitates and tunes the transduction process. Any disorder of the afferent division could result in findings similar to those shown by patients with auditory neuropathy. This "cochlear afferent disorder" could then be distinguished from the more common "cochlear efferent disorder" characterized by absent OAES and ABRs with normal morphology but elevated thresholds. Because almost all afferent nerve fibers are activated via the inner hair cells, pathologic processes specifically affecting the inner hair cells, the synapse between these cells, or both and the dendrites of the auditory nerve could also lead to a severe reduction in afferent activity (see Chapter 4 by Harrison in this book). Nevertheless, we feel that the most common pathophysiology for a cochlear afferent disorder, particularly in adults, is a neuropathy affecting the afferent nerve fibers and our discussion of this type of pathophysiology follows.

NEUROPATHY OF THE AUDITORY NERVE

The afferent auditory nerve fibers are myelinated bipolar neurons with their cell bodies in the spiral ganglion. Type I neurons innervate inner hair cells and comprise 95% of the afferent fibers. Between 10 and 30 Type I neurons synapse with a single inner hair cell providing optimal circumstance for synchrony of firing in this population. Type II neurons, which are small relative to the Type I, innervate outer hair cells and comprise the remaining 5% of the spiral ganglion population. Each Type II neuron makes contact with many outer hair cells, an arrangement not optimal for neural synchrony (Ryugo, 1992). The myelin in the distal portion of the auditory nerve derives from Schwann cells, the cells that provide myelin for the peripheral nerves. The myelin in the proximal portion of the nerve after it passes through the arachnoid to enter the brain stem derives from oligodendroglia, the cells providing the myelin for central nervous system axons. The boundary between the two types of myelin occurs as the auditory nerve passes through the dura/arachnoid near the cochlear nucleus. Auditory nerve fibers number approximately 30,000 in humans, and the axonal diameters are approximately twice that of the dendritic diameters (Spoendlin & Schrott, 1988). In adults, estimates of the axon diameters range from 0.5 to 11 micrometers (Natout, Terr, Linthicum, & House, 1987; Spoendlin & Schrott, 1988). Most of the fibers have diameters of approximately 3 μm. This relative uniformity of diameter and the resultant uniformity of conduction velocities favor synchrony of discharge among these fibers. Peripheral sensory nerves vary considerably more in size, ranging between 0.5 and 20 μm.

Neuropathies may be caused by a primary demyelination or by an axonal disease. The classification is ultimately based on histological examination of the affected nerves, but surface recordings the nerve conduction velocity and amplitude of nerve action potentials are often related to the histologic findings. In the case of the auditory nerve, histologic studies can only be done on postmortem examination of the temporal bone or the brain stem at the point of entry of the auditory nerve. For neuropathies of the peripheral nervous system, a biopsy of a small portion of a sensory nerve, such as the sural nerve, can be taken from the patient in the clinic.

Electrodiagnostic studies (nerve conduction studies and electromyography) can provide a functional categorization for the type of neuropathy (Kimura, 1989). Understanding how these electrodiagnostic studies might indicate the pathophysiology requires a brief review of how action potentials are conducted along nerve fibers and how they are recorded at a distance.

The conduction of action potentials along myelinated and unmyelinated nerve fibers can be illustrated by examining what happens when a myelinated fiber becomes unmyelinated (Bostock, 1993; Waxman, 1996). The distance that the action potential travels before it becomes too small to initiate another action potential will vary inversely with the current draining through the axonal membrane. A myelinated nerve fiber has a much greater membrane resistance than an unmyelinated fiber. The greater membrane resistance causes less current drain. The action potential can therefore travel a greater distance before it needs to be regenerated, and the conduction velocity is faster. A train of Schwann cells or oligodendroglial cells surround the axon with myelin, leaving between the adjacent boundaries of the cells a small region called a node of Ranvier where the axon is unmyelinated. These regions of the axon contain a high concentration of the voltage-dependent sodium ion-channels needed to generate an action potential. An action potential initiated in the terminal dendrite will spread rapidly along a myelinated fiber, reactivating itself at each node of Ranvier (Figure 5–1, top). Because the action potential effectively "jumps" from one node to the next (or from one node to another several nodes away), its progress is described as "saltatory" (from the Latin *saltare*, to jump). If the myelin thickness were reduced by disease, the resistance across the membrane would decrease so that the action potential does not spread as far before requiring regeneration, and the conduction velocity is slowed. If the Schwann cell and its myelin layers were acutely lost, the impulses would be unlikely to be conducted through the demyelinated region because few ion channels exist in the newly bared axon. Thus, the action potential cannot activate the subsequent node of Ranvier resulting in a conduction block (Figure 5–1, middle). With time, new ion channels may develop in the demyelinated region and the axon may again conduct impulses but at a slow velocity characteristic of unmyelinated axons (Figure 5–1, bottom). When the impulse reaches a zone of normal myelin, saltatory conduction is again possible, and conduction velocity is speeded.

These demyelinated fibers function abnormally in ways other than their slowed velocity (Waxman, 1996). First, they do not conduct rapid trains of action potentials very well. High discharge rates occur normally in response to intense acoustic stimuli, contributing to the appreciation of loudness and mediating reflex activation of middle ear muscles. Acoustic middle ear muscle reflexes are typically absent in subjects with auditory neuropathy, and the mechanism may be the failure of auditory nerve fibers to develop sufficiently high discharge rates to activate the motor neurons of the stapedius muscle. Second, demyelinated fibers are sensitive to increases in temperature and may develop conduction block. In this regard, we have reported two patients with the clinical picture of auditory neuropathy who have a temperature-sensitive hearing loss (Starr et al., 1998). Third, demyelinated axons become sensitive to mechanical stimulation. The location of the auditory nerve fibers protects them from any mechanical sensitivity, and this characteristic probably plays no role in the symptoms of auditory neuropathy. Fourth, demyelinated fibers may display ephaptic transmission ("cross-talk") between fibers, with one active fiber setting off discharges in adjacent fibers. If this were to occur in the auditory nerve, there might be severe distortion in the coding of complex sounds like speech.

Figure 5–2 illustrates sensory nerve action potentials in individual fibers and the resulting compound nerve action potential, which can be recorded by surfaces electrodes in the clinic. A primary demyelinating neuropathy is characterized by a slowing of conduction velocity. If the

Normal

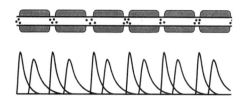

Conduction
Block

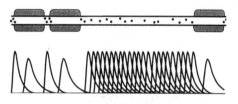

Demyelination
with Slowing

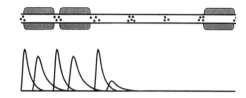

Figure 5–1. This is a diagrammatic representation of what occurs when a nerve fiber becomes demyelinated. The upper part of the figure shows a longitudinal section through a normally myelinated fiber. The sausage-shaped gray regions are the myelin sheath. The dark dots are the voltage-sensitive sodium channels that are concentrated at the nodes of Ranvier. Below the fiber is shown the action potential, represented stroboscopically as it is conducted along the axon. The amplitude of the action potential falls off a little as it spreads along the myelinated region of the axon, but it is still sufficiently large when it reaches the next node of Ranvier to activate the sodium channels and thereby regenerate itself. The central part of the figure shows what happens when the myelin is removed. The action potential falls off much more rapidly because of the reduced membrane resistance and cannot reach any excitable region of the axon with sufficient amplitude to regenerate itself. Conduction block ensues. The bottom part of the figure shows what happens when sodium channels diffuse into the bare axon. The action potential can now regenerate itself, but this occurs over much shorter distances than when the axon was myelinated and the conduction velocity is therefore very slow.

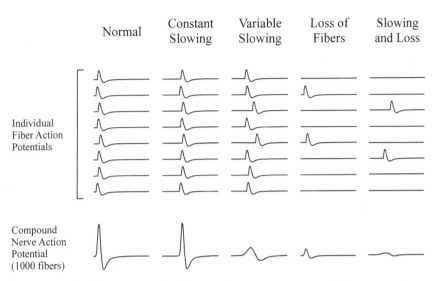

Figure 5–2. This figure was derived from a simple computer model that summed up the action potentials from 1,000 individual fibers (eight of which are shown) in a nerve. The velocity of the fibers could be consistently or variably slowed (second and third column). The fourth column shows what occurs when only one in five of the fibers remain. The fifth column represents a combination of the pathology shown in columns three and four.

demyelination affects all the fibers of a peripheral nerve to a similar degree, each fiber will be similarly slowed down, and the amplitude of the compound action potentials would be unaffected despite severe slowing of the conduction velocity (Figure 5–2, second column). If the amount of slowing varies from one fiber to the next, the amplitude of the compound action potentials becomes small and broadened (Figure 5–2, third column). In some instances, demyelination at a particular point may be sufficient to prevent conduction across the demyelinated zone (a conduction block), and no compound nerve action potential distal to the conduction block will be produced. Subjects with multiple sclerosis, a myelin disorder affecting axons within the central nervous system, can have demyelinated plaques in the brain stem auditory pathways. Changes in the ABR reflect the site(s) of demyelination so that ABR components generated distal to the zone of demyelination are of normal latency and amplitude, whereas components generated central to the zone of demyelination are delayed in latency and their amplitudes are typically reduced (Chiappa, 1997; Picton, 1990), compatible with variable slowing (Figure 5–2, third column). Occasionally wave V is delayed but of normal amplitude compatible with a constant slowing in the different fibers (Figure 5–2, second column). The central portion of the auditory nerve can be affected by a plaque producing an auditory neuropathy with wave I, the component generated by the peripheral portion of the 8th nerve, being the only remaining ABR constituent.

An axonal neuropathy is characterized by relatively normal conduction velocity and reduced amplitude of the compound nerve action potentials. The nerve fibers function normally in terms of the speed of conduction but are reduced in number (Figure 5–2, fourth column). Maximum rates of discharge are not affected to the same extent as in demyelinating neuropathies (Kuwabara et al., 1999).

Because the axon depends on the cell body for its sustenance, axonal neuropathies often will be most evident the farther one goes from the cell body. This can lead to a "dying back" of the distal processes. This is prominent in axonal neuropathies but is also apparent in any neuropathy because the longest fibers are most susceptible to pathology. The longest cochlear nerve fibers are those going to the apex of the cochlea, which is responsible for low frequencies (Figure 5–3, L). The shortest fibers are those going to the second half of the first cochlear turn, which is responsible for the middle frequencies (Figure 5–3, M). Those going to the initial

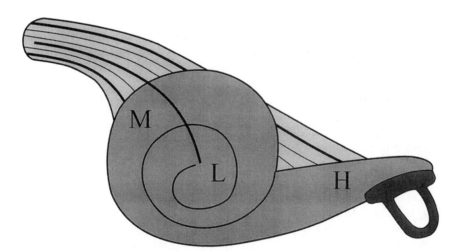

Figure 5–3. This figure shows the afferent innervation of the left cochlea viewed from an anterolateral perspective. The snail-shaped cochlea would be protruding outward. The fibers innervating the apical regions of the cochlea, and carrying low-frequency information (L), have the longest intra-cochlear course and wind up in the center of the cochlear nerve. The fibers innervating the high-frequency region (H) of the cochlea near the stapes also have a longer course than the fibers innervating the mid-frequency region (M).

part of the basal turn near the stapes, which is responsible, for the high frequencies (Figure 5–3, H) have lengths between these extremes. If the auditory neuropathy were to exhibit a dying back pathophysiology, the audiogram would show a low-frequency hearing loss. This type of audiogram is common in auditory neuropathy subjects (see Chapter 2 by Sininger and Oba).

In an axonal peripheral neuropathy, there is usually a greater abnormality of the muscles than in a demyelinating neuropathy, where the remaining axons might still maintain some trophic interaction with the muscles that they innervate. Patients with hereditary demyelinating disorders often show normal muscle activity despite severe slowing of their nerve conduction velocities. If the auditory neuropathy were axonal and if it involved the efferent fibers as well as the afferent fibers, one might expect some decrease in the function of the external hair cells. We might therefore speculate that the progressive hearing loss with threshold elevation and loss of OAEs that develops in some patients with auditory neuropathy might be more likely due to an axonal rather than demyelinating neuropathy. This suggestion requires that the neuropathic process also involve the efferent system.

The axon and its myelin sheath are intimately related, and one cannot exist well without the other. The boundary between axonal and demyelinating neuropathies is therefore not always as precise as we have suggested. An axonal neuropathy is often accompanied by histologic evidence of focal areas of secondary demyelination and remyelination, and demyelinating neuropathies may also have histologic evidence of axonal loss. These concomitant pathologies become more evident as the neuropathy persists. In a hereditary form of auditory neuropathy due to a genetic change at 8q24 (Butinar et al., 1999), there is a disorder of a signaling protein (Kalaydjieva et al., 2000) between Schwann cells and axons affecting a disruption of both elements (King et al., 1999). The effect of combined axonal and demyelinating disorders on auditory nerve fibers is schematically represented in the last column of Figure 5–2.

RELATIONSHIP OF PATHOPHYSIOLOGY TO SIGNS AND SYMPTOMS

The two major physiologic changes accompanying neuropathies of the auditory nerve would be (a) disruption of temporal synchrony of the auditory input due to demyelination and (b) reduction of the number of fibers conducting to the central pathways due to axonal loss. The two processes could also occur together.

The consequences of altered neural synchrony might account for some of the cardinal features of auditory neuropathy. First, loss of synchrony would disrupt the time locking of auditory nerve responses to repeated signals so that an averaged ABR could not be detected. Second, altered neural synchrony could selectively affect auditory perceptions dependent on temporal cues (gap detection, localization, masking level difference, amplitude modulation detection, low-frequency pitch discrimination; see Starr et al., 1991; Zeng et al., 1999; Zeng et al., Chapter 8 in this book). Third, the prominence of impaired low-frequency hearing in auditory neuropathy subjects could be related to altered synchrony essential for encoding low-frequency auditory signals. The loss of neural synchrony alone, however, could not account for the absence of middle ear muscle and olivocochlear reflexes in this disorder.

The consequences of reduced neural input could also account for some of the features of auditory neuropathy. First, ABRs would be absent if the input were sufficiently reduced. In persons with normal hearing, however, ABRs can still be detected when the signal intensity is close to hearing threshold, suggesting that decreased input alone is not sufficient to account for the absence of ABRs found in most subjects with auditory neuropathy.

Second, the loss of acoustic reflexes (middle ear muscles and olivocochlear bundle activation of OHC) could be secondary to axonal loss. These reflexes are evoked using suprathreshold signals that activate a large number of auditory nerves, and this may not be possible with axonal loss.

Third, auditory temporal processes could also be affected by a decrease of input. Some of the behavioral measures of temporal processes such as gap detection are significantly elevated when signal intensity is reduced, approaching values seen in some auditory neuropathy subjects.

We can perceive time structures at rates faster than the maximum rate at which a single nerve fiber can discharge (Viemeister & Plack, 1993). A possible explanation for this is the "volley theory" of hearing (Wever, 1949), which proposes that multiple neurons can encode a rapid temporal waveform even though any one could not fire as rapidly as necessary to code the waveform by itself. For example, a 500-Hz tone can be encoded by five neurons each firing at 100 Hz provided that each of the five neurons fires on a different cycle from the others. If the volley theory is correct, then a loss of neurons (axonal neuropathy) might cause as much disruption in the encoding of rapid temporal patterns as the desynchronization of neurons (demyelinating neuropathy). Thus, axonal loss, demyelination, or a combination of both can disrupt the encoding of rapid temporal patterns. Most subjects with auditory neuropathy have a low-frequency or flat hearing loss with a moderate threshold elevation. Low-frequency tones near threshold may be encoded by phase synchronization rather than a change in rate of discharges (Rose, Hind, Anderson, & Brugge, 1971). The two processes are not significantly different for enabling the identification that a sound has occurred, however (Johnson, 1980). Thus, although a disorder of synchronization would clearly decrease discrimination among low frequencies, it may not necessarily affect the detection of near-threshold tones (Delgutte, 1996). The low-frequency hearing loss in many persons with auditory neuropathy could be explained by loss of afferent input from the apical portion of the cochlea (axonal) or loss of synchronization of this input (demyelination). At middle and high frequencies, the elevation of thresholds could not be due to desynchronization of neural inputs. Experimental animal studies involving lesions of inner hair cells (see Chapter 4 by Harrison in this book) or auditory nerve (Zheng et al., 1999) has shown that the threshold of single units in the central auditory pathway can remain normal despite these lesions. A recent study by Salvi, Wang, and Ding (2000) has documented that auditory cortical responses in animals with lesions of inner hair cells have normal or heightened intensity functions compatible with reorganization of the central auditory system. Because it may not be possible to relate the threshold change in subjects with auditory neuropathy to afferent damage, we suggest that a loss of the efferent olivo-cochlear bundle system might affect tuning sensitivities in a manner sufficient to produce the moderate threshold elevation found in these subjects.

NEUROPATHOLOGY OF AUDITORY NEUROPATHY

We have examined the sural nerve in six individuals with auditory neuropathy and a concomitant peripheral neuropathy (see Starr, Chapter 3 in this book, for a photomicrograph of one of the biopsies). The histology of the sural nerve in one subject was consistent with an axonal neuropathy affecting a loss of large myelinated fibers. Three other subjects had axonal loss with evidence of secondary demyelination and remyelination of the remaining fibers. The biopsy from one of the three is shown in Chapter 3 of this book. Only one of these two subjects had slowed nerve conduction. The final two subjects' sural nerve biopsies showed extensive loss of both axons and myelin with only few remaining fibers still present (see Butinar et al., 1999, for the histology of one of the subjects). The other patient with extensive loss of axons and myelin in the sural nerve was age 77 at the time the sural nerve was sampled at autopsy. This patient had an adult late-onset hereditary sensory-motor neuropathy (HSMN) beginning at age 40, and a hearing loss developing 10 years later. The disorder was inherited in a dominant manner, and DNA analysis of affected family members showed a duplication disorder on the MPZ gene on chromosome 1. The patient died this year, and the auditory and sural nerves showed a loss of nerve fibers with the extent of the nerve loss being considerably more advanced in the sural than in the auditory nerve. The

Auditory Nerve

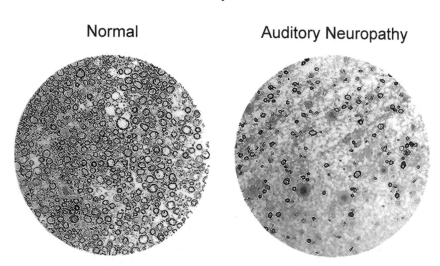

Figure 5–4. Photomicrographs (enlarged 325×) of a cross section of the auditory nerve in a patient with hereditary sensory-motor neuropathy (HSMN) and deafness who died at age 77 and an aged-match subject who died of an illness not involving the central nervous system. There is a marked reduction in the number of auditory nerve fibers in the HSMN patient. The sural nerve in the patient also showed axonal loss with evidence of demyelination and remyelination.

photomicrograph in Figure 5–4 contains a portion of the auditory nerve close to the brain stem in the patient (right) and an age-matched control subject (left). There is a striking loss of nerve fibers in the auditory nerve in the auditory neuropathy patient compared with the control subject. If the pathologic process followed a time course similar to that defined in sural nerve, the loss would have first involved large fibers. Experimental studies demonstrate that the large auditory nerve fibers are distinguished by high spontaneous discharge rates (Gleich & Wilson, 1993), fast conduction velocities, and low thresholds (Liberman, 1982). These large fiber characteristics may be relevant for defining some of the attributes of the hearing loss of subjects with auditory neuropathy.

To summarize, a neuropathic disorder of the auditory and peripheral nerves occurs in the majority of adults with a syndrome of auditory neuropathy. When biopsy tissue is available, pathology of sural nerves showed loss of large myelinated fibers and evidence of both primary and secondary demyelination. The neuropathology of one auditory nerve sampled at postmortem expressed features of axonal loss. We consider the pathophysiology of the disorder to include both impairments of neural synchrony of auditory nerve fibers secondary to demyelination and a loss of the number of functioning fibers secondary to axonal loss. An unresolved question that will be addressed below is the physiologic bases of "auditory neuropathy" in infants and children who do not have evidence of a peripheral neuropathy. Do these children have an isolated neuropathic disorder of the auditory nerve, or are cochlear elements distal to the nerve (synapse or inner hair cells) affected?

SYNAPTIC DISORDERS

A disorder of the synapse between inner hair cells and auditory nerve dendrites would certainly affect auditory nerve activity, perhaps in a manner that would cause the clinical disorder of "auditory neuropathy." The inner hair cell has specialized anatomic structures at its base that presumably are involved in the storage and release of neurotransmitter(s), which act on receptor sites on the dendrites of the auditory nerve and cause the generation of action potentials. Synaptic disorders can be presynaptic (e.g., impaired inner hair cell functions) or postsynaptic (e.g., altered receptors on auditory nerve dendrite). We are not aware of diagnostic procedures that can clearly distinguish between pre- and postsynaptic disorders.

The effect of stimulus rate on ABR in healthy subjects has been proposed as reflecting synaptic changes (Pratt & Sohmer, 1976). The amplitude of the ABR beginning with wave I becomes reduced, and latency is prolonged as stimulus rate increases. The mechanisms for this effect may be presynaptic affecting depletion of neurotransmitter stores or postsynaptic involving a depolarizing block of dendrites.

A well-studied model of a synaptic disorder in humans is myasthenia gravis, which affects the neuromuscular junction. In myasthenia gravis, receptor sites on the muscle membrane are inactivated by autoantibodies limiting the number of binding sites for the neurotransmitter, acetylcholine, released by the motor nerve terminals. Patients with myasthenia gravis complain of fatigue that can be provoked by repetitive muscle activity. Electrodiagnostic studies of the peripheral nerve and muscle in this disorder show a decline of amplitude of motor potentials to repetitive nerve stimulation similar in style to the rate effects on wave I of the ABR in healthy subjects.

Some patients with auditory neuropathy have a marked sensitivity of the ABR to stimulus rates compatible with a rate-sensitive synaptic disorder. We found three subjects (Figure 5–5) with absent ABRs at stimulus rates of 20/s but clear wave Vs at slow rates of stimulation (11 and 3/s). Note in Figure 5–5 that the outer CM in the beginning of the averaged responses, which is generated by the hair cells, did not change in amplitude with stimulus rate. A stimulus rate of 20/s should not stress synaptic

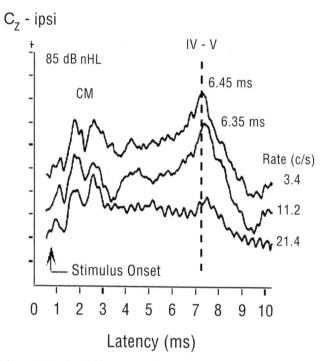

Figure 5–5. Cochlear microphonic (CM) and auditory brain stem response (ABR) potentials in response to clicks as a function of stimulus rate. Note the clear CM in all traces and the reduction of wave V of the ABR and the increase in latency as click rate changed from 11.2/sec to 21.4/sec. The amplitude scale is 0.3 uV/division.

function in normal subjects, and it is a rate customarily used in many facilities to test the ABR. Rate effects as described might also occur in a demyelinating neuropathy.

The use of interventional medicines to facilitate or increase neurotransmitters for the treatment of neurological disorders is now common. Disordered synaptic function may be the basis for certain instances of hearing loss we call "auditory neuropathy." Identification of a transmitter or receptor impairment in these instances might lead to effective pharmacologic therapy for these patients.

INNER HAIR CELL DISORDERS

Animal studies of Harrison (see Chapter 4 in this book and Harrison, 1998) are instructive showing that anoxia and toxic agents such as carboplatinum selectively affect inner hair cells to impair auditory nerve function. The loss of inner hair cells effectively removes the transduction process including the release of neurotransmitters that activate auditory nerve dendrites. It is not yet clear whether the dendrites are also directly affected by these situations as both inner hair cells and the auditory nerve can degenerate in animal studies. An excess of neurotransmitters can also effect an attenuation of auditory nerve activity. Infusion of synaptic agonists in the cochlea of animals is accompanied by a loss of function of auditory nerve fibers (Zheng et al., 1999). Thus, both excess and loss of synaptic functions can disrupt auditory nerve input. The relationship between these animal models of peripheral auditory dysfunction and the human condition of auditory neuropathy merits further investigation. We would expect that some of the neonatal exposures to anoxia and toxic factors accompanying hyperbilirubinemia are likely acting at the inner hair cell–synapse regions.

SUMMARY

The condition called auditory neuropathy is likely a group of disorders affecting the function of (a) auditory nerve directly (neuropathic disorder), (b) inner hair cells, and (c) synapses between auditory nerve and inner hair cells. Methods for distinguishing these pathologies are unclear. Chapter 1 by Kraus on historical perspectives provides insight as to how scientists and clinicians grapple with uncertainty, waxing between denial and insight. Eventually we will understand the condition of auditory neuropathy in detail and will have therapies for some of the varieties. Time is on our side.

Acknowledgments: Portions of this work were supported by the National Institute on Deafness and Other Communicative Disorders Grant No. R01-DC02618. Dr. Ronald Kim, neuropathologist at the University of California, Irvine, was instrumental to the neuropathologic analysis and to sections in this chapter.

REFERENCES

Berlin, C. I., Bordelon, J., St. John, P., Wilensky, D., Hurley, A., Kluka, E., & Hood, L. J. (1998). Reversing click polarity may uncover auditory neuropathy in infants. *Ear and Hearing, 19,* 37–47.
Bostock, H. (1993). Impulse propagation in experimental neuropathy. In P. J. Dyck, P. K. Thomas, J. W. Griffin, P. A. Low, & J. F. Poduslo, (Eds.), *Peripheral neuropathy* (pp. 109–120). Philadelphia: Saunders.

Butinar, D., Zidar, J., Leonardis, L., Popovic, M., Kalaydjieva, L., Angelicheva, D., Sininger, Y., Keats, B., & Starr, A. (1999). Hereditary auditory, vestibular, motor, and sensory neuropathy in a Slovenian Roma (Gypsy) kindred. *Annals of Neurology, 46,* 36–44.

Chiappa, K. H. (1997). *Evoked potentials in clinical medicine* (4th ed.) Philadelphia: Lippincott.

Delgutte, B. (1996). Physiological models for basic auditory percepts. In H. L. Hawkins, T. A. McMullen, A. N. Popper, & R. R. Fay (Eds.), *Auditory computation* (pp. 157–220). New York: Springer-Verlag.

Gleich, O., & Wilson, S. (1993). The diameters of guinea pig auditory nerve fibres: Distribution and correlation with spontaneous rate. *Hearing Research, 71,* 69–79.

Harrison, R. V. (1998). An animal model of auditory neuropathy. *Ear and Hearing, 19,* 355–361.

Johnson, D. H. (1980). The relationship between spike rate and synchrony in responses of auditory nerve-fibers to single tones. *Journal of the Acoustical Society of America, 68,* 1115–1122.

Kalaydjieva, L., Gresham, D., Gooding, R., Heather, L., Baas, F., de Jonge, R., Blechschmidt, K., Angelicheva, D., Chandler, D., Worsley, P., Rosenthal, A., King, R. H., & Thomas, P. K. (2000). N-myc downstream-regulated gene 1 is mutated in hereditary motor and sensory neuropathy-Lom. *American Journal of Human Genetics, 67,* 47–58.

Kimura, J. (1989). *Electrodiagnosis in diseases of nerve and muscle: Principles and practice* (2nd ed.) Philadelphia: F. A. Davis.

King, R. H., Tournev, I., Colomer, J., Merlini, L., Kalaydjieva, L., & Thomas, P. K. (1999). Ultrastructural changes in peripheral nerve in hereditary motor and sensory neuropathy-Lom. *Neuropathology and Applied Neurobiology, 25,* 306–312.

Kuwabara, S., Nakajima, Y., Hattori, T., Toma, S., Mizobuchi, K., & Ogawara, K. (1999). Activity-dependent excitability changes in chronic inflammatory demyelinating polyneuropathy: A microneurographic study. *Muscle and Nerve, 22,* 899–904

Liberman, M. C. (1982). Single-neuron labeling in the cat auditory nerve. *Science, 216,* 1239–1241.

Natout, M. A. Y., Terr, L. I., Linthicum, F. H., House, W. F. (1987). Topography of vestibulocochlear nerve fibers in the posterior cranial fossa. *Laryngoscope, 97,* 954–958.

Picton, T. W. (1990). Auditory evoked potentials. In D. D. Daly & T. A. Pedley (Eds.), *Current practice of clinical electroencephalography* (2nd ed., pp. 625–678). New York: Raven Press.

Pratt, H., & Sohmer, H. (1976). Intensity and rate functions of cochlear and brainstem evoked responses to click stimuli in man. *Archives of Oto-Rhino-Laryngology, 12,* 85–92.

Probst, R., Lonsbury-Martin, B. L., & Martin, G. K. (1991). A review of otoacoustic emissions. *Journal of the Acoustical Society of America, 89,* 2027–2067.

Rose, J. E., Hind, J. E., Anderson, D. J., & Brugge, J. F. (1971). Some effects of stimulus intensity on response of auditory nerve fibers in the squirrel monkey. *Journal of Neurophsyiology, 34,* 685–699.

Ryugo, D. K. (1992). The auditory nerve: Peripheral innervations, cell body morphology, and central projections. In D. R. Webster, A. N. Popper, & R. Fay (Eds.),

The mammalian auditory pathway: Neuroanatomy (pp. 23–65). New York: Springer-Verlag.

Salvi, R. J., Wang, J., & Ding, D. (2000). Auditory plasticity and hyperactivity following cochlear damage. *Hearing Research, 147,* 261–274.

Spoendlin, H., & Schrott, A. (1988). The spiral ganglion and innervation of the human organ of Corti. *Acta Oto-Laryngologica (Stockholm), 105,* 403–410.

Starr, A., & Don, M. (1988). Brain potentials evoked by acoustic stimuli. In Picton, T. W. (Ed.), *Handbook of electroencephalography and clinical neurophysiology. Human event-related potentials* (revised series, Vol. 3, pp. 97–157). Amsterdam: Elsevier.

Starr, A., McPherson, D., Patterson, J., Don, M., Luxford, W. M., Shannon, R., Sininger, Y. S., Tonokawa, L. T., & Waring, M. (1991). Absence of both auditory evoked potentials and auditory percepts dependent on timing cues. *Brain, 114,* 1157–1180.

Starr, A., Picton, T. W., Sininger, Y., Hood, L. J., & Berlin, C. I. (1996). Auditory neuropathy. *Brain, 119,* 741–753.

Starr, A., Sininger, Y. S., Winter, M., Derebery, J., Oba, S., & Michalewski, H. (1998). Transient deafness due to temperature-sensitive auditory neuropathy. *Ear and Hearing, 19,* 169–179.

Starr, A., Sininger, Y., Nguyen, T., Michalewski, H., Oba, S., & Abdala, C. (in press). Cochlear receptor (microphonic and summating potentials, otoacoustic emissions) and auditory pathway (auditory brainstem potentials) activity in auditory neuropathy. *Ear and Hearing.*

Viemeister, N. F., & Plack, C. J. (1993). Time analysis. In W. A. Yost, A. N. Popper, & R. R. Fay (Eds.), *Human psychophysics* (pp. 116–154). New York: Springer-Verlag.

Waxman, S. G. (1996). Pathophysiology of demyelinated and remyelinated axons. In S. D. Cook (Ed.), *Handbook of multiple sclerosis* (2nd ed., pp. 257–293). New York: Marcel Dekker.

Wever, E. G. (1949). *Theory of hearing.* New York: Wiley.

Zeng, F. G., Oba, S., Garde, S., Sininger, Y., & Starr, A. (1999). Temporal and speech processing deficits in auditory neuropathy. *Neuroreport, 10,* 3429–3435.

Zheng, X. Y., Salvi, R. J., McFadden, S. L., Ding, D. L., & Henderson, D. (1999). Recovery of kainic acid excitotoxicity in chinchilla cochlea. *Annals of the New York Academy of Science, 884,* 255–269.

6

Anatomy of the Human
Cochlea and Auditory Nerve

Jean K. Moore and Fred H. Linthicum, Jr.

Published descriptions of subjects with auditory neuropathy (Doyle, Sininger, & Starr, 1998; Starr et al., 1991; Starr, Picton, Sininger, Hood, & Berlin, 1996) present an enigma, in that some of the commonly used signs of auditory function appear completely normal, whereas others are distinctly abnormal or even absent. Cochlear microphonic potentials are normal in form and amplitude. Otoacoustic emissions are also present but are not suppressed by stimulation of the contralateral ear. Most notably, brain stem auditory evoked potentials are distorted or missing. Even with high-intensity click or tone stimuli, no identifiable components of the short-latency potentials can be detected, but the middle and, more commonly, long-latency evoked potentials can be seen in some of these patients. Can this physiologic profile be related to the structure of the peripheral auditory system, namely, the cochlea and auditory nerve? The goal of this chapter is to review the anatomy of the peripheral auditory system in relation to the functions used in diagnosis of auditory neuropathy and to consider the implications of the functional deficits for the location of the pathologic process.

OVERVIEW OF THE PERIPHERAL AUDITORY SYSTEM

An overview of the lower auditory system can be gained from a radiologic image of a human head at the level of the brain stem (Figure 6–1). The section passes through the cochlea within the petrous portion of the temporal bone. The section also shows the emergence of the auditory nerve from the internal acoustic meatus (porus acusticus) on the medial side of the petrous pyramid. From this point, the nerve passes across the

83

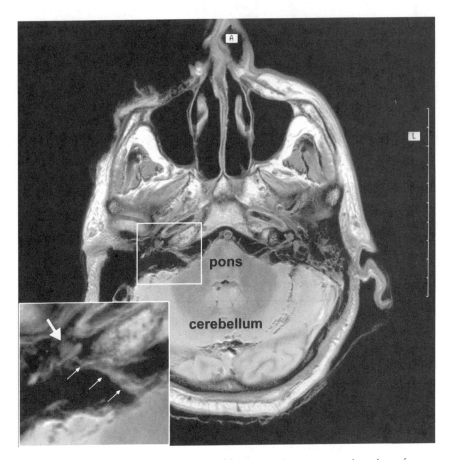

Figure 6–1. A radiologic image obtained by magnetic resonance imaging of a cadaver head. The bar on the right side of the image is a centimeter scale. The bony defect on the left side of the head shows that it had undergone a translabyrinthine surgical procedure. This transaxial section passes through the cochlea within the petrous portion of temporal bone. From the cochlea, the auditory nerve passes across the intradural space to the brain stem. At this level, the brain stem is represented by the pons and cerebellum. *Inset:* A higher power view of the cochlea (large arrow) and auditory nerve (small arrows). A = anterior; L = lateral.

cerebrospinal fluid-filled intradural space to the point where it enters the brain stem. It is apparent that the intradural segment of the nerve constitutes a considerable portion of its total length. The nerve enters the lower pons and terminates in the cochlear nuclei, which are not visible in this image. At higher power (Figure 6–1, inset), it is possible to see the turns of the cochlea from base to apex and the spiraling of the fascicles of axons in the nerve.

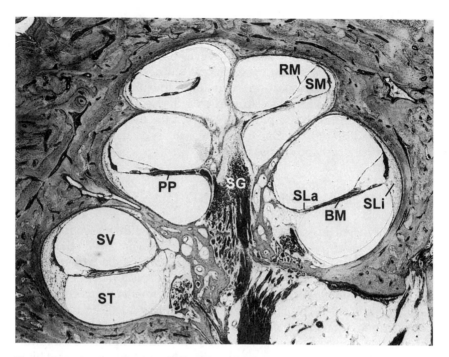

Figure 6–2. A microphotograph showing the major structural features of the human cochlea. Hematoxylin-eosin stain. BM = basilar membrane; PP = peripheral processes; RM = Reissner's membrane; SG = spiral ganglion; SLa = spiral lamina; SLi = spiral ligament; SM = scala media; ST = scala tympani; SV = scala vestibuli.

The first stage of hearing involves a purely mechanical transmission of acoustic energy from the structures of the middle ear and thus does not generate recordable potentials. The structures involved in mechanical transmission within the cochlea are shown in Figure 6–2, a horizontal section through the cochlea from apex to base in the same plane as the image in Figure 6–1. The cochlea is a coiled, fluid-filled tube that is divided along its length into two compartments by a flexible partition. This partition, the basilar membrane, is suspended between the shelf-like spiral lamina medially and the spiral ligament on the lateral wall of the cochlea. The fluid space on the apical side of the partition is known as the scala vestibuli, and that on the basal side is termed the scala tympani. Both compartments are filled with perilymph, which resembles extracellular fluid in that it is high in sodium and low in potassium. The two scalae are continuous with each other at the extreme apical end of the cochlea. When acoustic stimuli impart vibratory motion to the tympanic membrane and ossicles, the footplate of the stapes creates a piston-like driving force on the oval window, opening into the extreme basal end of the scala vestibuli. The resulting pressure waves within the perilymph cause an undulation of the basilar membrane, which is known as the traveling wave. Because the basilar membrane varies in width and stiffness along its length, the shape of the traveling wave and the point of maximum displacement of the membrane varies from base to apex with the frequency of the stimulus in cycles per second. These properties impart the first level of frequency specificity and tuning of cochlear elements, an aspect of cochlear function that is beyond the scope of this chapter.

COCHLEAR HAIR CELLS AND TRANSDUCTION

The sensory elements of the cochlea are contained within a separate fluid compartment, the scala media or cochlear duct, which rests on the lateral end of the basilar membrane (Figure 6–2). The scala media is bounded on its basal side by the basilar membrane and on its apical side by Reissner's membrane. A higher power view of this compartment and its contents is seen in Figure 6–3A. The lateral wall of the cochlear duct is formed by the stria vascularis, a cellular layer on the surface of the spiral ligament. Through the action of the stria vascularis, the endolymphatic fluid of the scala media is held in a unique ionic composition of low sodium and high potassium. Maintenance of the ionic difference between perilymph and endolymph is a vital factor in cochlear function.

The transformation of mechanical to bioelectric energy occurs within the organ of Corti. Although the process involves the activity of several types of specialized support cells, it is primarily a function of cochlear hair cells. The general orientation of the single row of inner hair cells and three rows of outer hair cells is shown diagrammatically in Figure 6–3B. The distinguishing feature of hair cells, as their name implies, is the array of thin processes, the stereocilia, on their upper surface. The organization of the stereociliary bundles differs to some degree for inner and outer hair cells. In man, as in other mammals, stereocilia on inner hair cells are arranged in a shallow U curve, whereas they have a more precise geometry in outer hair cells, forming a V- or W-shaped bundle (Wright, 1981). In both types of hair cell, each stereociliary bundle is ordered in rows of increasing length from inner to outer within the U- or V-shaped array (Figure 6–3B). Overall length varies, with the tallest stereocilia located on hair cells at the cochlear apex. A greater range from short to long occurs in outer hair cells. Stereocilia in outer and inner hair cells are similar in being comprised of long actin filaments, organized into bundles and arrays by fimbrin (Flock, Bretscher, & Weber, 1982; Flock, Cheung, Flock, & Utter, 1981). The actin filaments extend through the rootlets of the stereocilia, anchoring them into the cuticular plate on the surface of the hair cell.

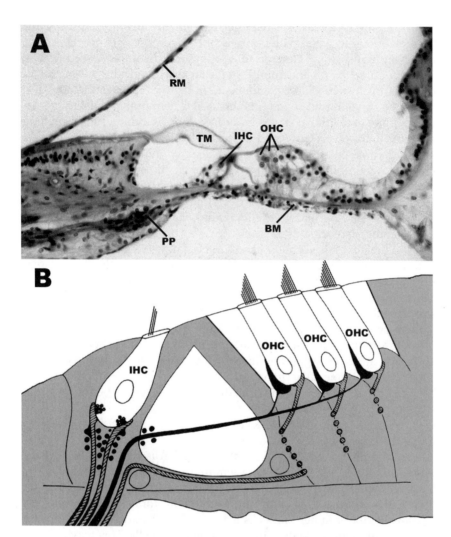

Figure 6–3. A: A high-power microphotograph of the scala media and organ of Corti. Hematoxylin-eosin stain. **B:** A diagrammatic representation of the organ of Corti and its innervation. Hair cells are illustrated in white and supporting structures in grey. Afferent nerves and terminals are shown in black, and efferent nerve fibers are cross-hatched. BM = basilar membrane; IHC = inner hair cells; OHC = outer hair cells; PP = peripheral processes; RM = Reissner's membrane; StV = stria vascularis; TM = tectorial membrane. (Adapted from Spoendlin, 1985.)

In Figure 6–3A, as is usual after fixation and histologic processing, the gelatinous tectorial membrane is not in contact with the hair cells; however, high-voltage electron micropsopy on thick tissue sections (Takasaka et al., 1983) has demonstrated that the tips of the tallest row of outer hair cell stereocilia are embedded in the tectorial membrane. Thus, when the traveling wave deflects the basilar membrane, causing motion of the organ of Corti that sits on its surface, there is a change in orientation of outer hair cells relative to the tectorial membrane. This results in a shearing force exerted on their stereociliary bundles. Because only the tallest row of outer hair cell stereocilia is attached to the tectorial membrane, the shearing force might be expected to deflect only this row. Electron microscopy reveals a series of cross-links within each bundle, however. The individual stereocilia are linked by fine filaments, with side-links joining stereocilia in the same row and tip-links connecting shorter rows to the next tallest row (Furness & Hackney, 1985; Pickles, Comis, & Osborne 1984). These side-to-side and row-to-row connections form a regular lattice and cause the bundle to move as a single unit when the tectorial membrane displaces the tallest row. Deflection toward the tallest row stretches the tip links, and deflection toward the shortest row releases tension on the links. Experiments in lower vertebrates (Hudspeth, 1989) have shown that deflection of the stereociliary bundle, with alternate stretching and relaxing of the fibrous links joining the individual stereocilia, activates molecular channels in the stereociliary membrane. This is believed to be the first step in transduction. Molecular labeling of single stereocilia provides evidence for a similar process in mammals because the attachment points of the links to the stereocilia are the sites of calcium influx (Denk, Holt, Shepherd, & Corey, 1995).

A continuing question in cochlear function is that the stereociliary bundles of inner hair cells do not seem to have a direct attachment to the tectorial membrane. It is possible that their sterociliary bundles may be deflected by viscous drag of the fluid in the subtectorial space. The process of transduction in inner hair cells is not well understood, but it appears that it is not identical to the process in outer hair cells. This may account for the fact that inner hair cell stereocilia are less anatomically specialized than those of outer hair cells.

Activity of hair cells during transduction appears to be reflected in the cochlear microphonic. This externally recordable potential was originally believed to be generated by the auditory nerve. It differs from neural potentials, however, in being less sensitive to temperature changes, blood supply, and anoxia. Furthermore, its latency does not change with stimulus intensity, and it remains in the presence of noise sufficient to mask the auditory stimulus. The assumption that the cochlear microphonic is produced by activity of hair cells is supported by its disappearance in guinea pigs whose hair cells had been destroyed by administration of the antibiotic kanamycin (Dallos & Cheatham, 1976). These experiments also demonstrated an imbalance in the contribution of inner and outer hair cells to the cochlear microphonic. On schedules of kanamycin administration that destroyed primarily inner hair cells, leaving an almost normal complement of outer hair cells, the cochlear microphonic was essentially normal. When only inner hair cells remained, the microphonic was only a small fraction of normal. The lack of contribution of inner hair cells to the cochlear microphonic was confirmed when direct intracellular recordings showed that their activity does not follow either basilar membrane displacement or the extracellularly recorded cochlear microphonic (Sellick & Russell, 1980). The current belief is that the cochlear microphonic is generated by hair cell activity, principally or exclusively that of outer hair cells, during the transduction process. The presence of a normal cochlear microphonic in subjects with auditory neuropathy suggests that their outer hair cell transduction process is functioning normally.

OUTER HAIR CELL MOTILITY

The evidence on generation of the cochlear microphonic potential by outer hair cells implies some functional specialization on their part. As previously mentioned, both inner and outer hair cells contain the contractile molecules actin and fimbrin in their stereocilia. Recent research has shown that outer hair cells have, in addition, an active contractile process in their cell bodies. Antibody labeling has demonstrated that outer hair cells contain a layer of actin filaments between the plasma membrane of the cell wall and the subsurface fenestrated cisternae. The cell plasma membrane and cisternae are also interconnected by regularly spaced pillars, resembling those seen in the contractile system of muscle fibers. Physiologic experiments on isolated, dissociated outer hair cells have shown that they slowly shorten when exposed to a solution that would induce contraction in a muscle fiber (Flock, Flock, & Ulfendahl, 1986). In addition, they undergo shortening or lengthening in a frequency-specific manner when stimulated by an electric current (Brownell, 1984; Brownell, Bader, Bertrand, & de Ribaupierre, 1985; Brundin, Flock, & Canlon, 1989). Recent research has identified the protein termed "prestin" as that responsible for the motor contractile function of the outer hair cell (Zheng et al., 2000). Prestin is not found in inner hair cells, which lack the specialized system of tubules and actin filaments in their cell wall and show no motile responses under the same conditions.

The importance of outer hair cell motility in the process of transduction was demonstrated when somatic motion was induced by deflection of the stereociliary bundle (Evans & Dallos, 1993). The somatic shape change is sensitive to the direction of displacement of the bundle (i.e., toward or away from the tallest rows) and is abolished if the active transduction process is blocked. Outer hair cell motility is generally believed to be the basis of the sharp tuning and low threshold in mammalian hearing, as shown by raised behavioral thresholds in the absence of outer hair cells (Ryan & Dallos, 1975). In addition, outer hair cells are believed to be the physical substrate of otoacoustic emissions, with active shape changes in outer hair cells providing mechanical feedback to the basilar membrane. Indirect evidence for a connection between outer hair cells and otoacoustic emissions comes from observations that conditions which weaken the subsurface contractile structures, such as exposure to salicylates, also abolish otoacoustic emissions (Brownell, 1990). Recent experiments provided a direct demonstration that outer hair cell contraction can cause motion of the basilar membrane. When outer hair cells in an isolated cochlea were stimulated by electrical current, the electrically driven hair cell length changes produced a degree of vibration of the basilar membrane comparable to what occurs during acoustic stimulation (Mammano & Ashmore, 1993). The process is termed "reverse transduction" because it reverses the usual sequence of events during audition. Outer hair cell length changes move the basilar membrane, which in turn produces pressure waves in perilymph, motion of the ossicles, and oscillation of the tympanic membrane. The vibration of the tympanic membrane results in audible sound being emitted from the ear. Thus, the presence of otoacoustic emissions, and that of a cochlear microphonic, implies normally functioning outer hair cells in subjects with auditory neuropathy.

EFFERENT INNERVATION OF THE COCHLEA

One type of cochlear innervation consists of efferent, or outgoing, axons, which originate in the brain stem, travel in the 8th nerve, and terminate on cochlear hair cells. In the human cochlea (Nadol, 1983a, 1983b), as in other mammalian species, the efferent terminals end most prominently on outer hair cell bodies (see Figure 6–3B). Because the principal neurotransmitter of the efferent system is acetylcholine, it is not surprising that outer hair cell motility is affected by application of this substance. The original experiments on outer hair cell motility (Brownell, 1984) showed that application of acetylcholine, as well as electric current, caused cellular shape changes. Later experiments (Sziklai, He, & Dallos, 1996) determined that application of acetylcholine to isolated outer hair cells interacts with electrical stimulation, increasing the magnitude and gain in motility. The effects disappeared if agents that block acetylcholine receptors were applied.

Investigations of the human cochlear efferent system indicate that it has the same cholinergic nature as that of other mammals. Early investigations (Ishi, Murakami, & Ballogh, 1967; Schuknecht, Churchill, &

Doran, 1959) showed the presence of axons and terminals labeled with an acetylcholine-related enzyme in relation to human hair cells. The same type of histochemical marking traced efferent axons leaving the human brain stem (Moore & Osen, 1979). Recently, immunolabeling for acetylcholine revealed the population of cholinergic neurons in the human superior olivary complex, which are the origin of the efferent, or olivocochlear, projections (Moore, Simmons, & Guan, 1999). The human efferent system is presumed to be the basis for the normal suppression of the amplitude of otoacoustic emissions by acoustic stimulation of the opposite ear, a process that activates olivocochlear neurons (Berlin et al., 1993b). Suppression of otoacoustic emissions by contralateral stimulation does not occur in subjects with auditory neuropathy (Berlin, Hood, Cecola, Jackson, & Szabo, 1993a), however, even though the contractile mechanism of their outer hair cells appears to be normal (see Hood and Berlin, Chapter 10, this volume).

THE AUDITORY NERVE AND AFFERENT CONDUCTION

The origins of the afferent nerve system, through which information is transmitted from the cochlea to the brain, are the synaptic terminals contacting the bases of the hair cells (see Figure 6–3B). These terminals, and the short length (approximately 100 microns) of unmyelinated process beyond them, are the dendritic (or information receiving) ends of cochlear neurons. As the fibers pass through the habenula perforata, a series of small apertures in the osseous spiral lamina, they become surrounded by a coating of myelin created by Schwann cells. The myelinated processes continue along the spiral lamina, bend slightly downward as they enter the modiolus, and reach their cells of origin in the spiral ganglion (Figure 6–4). The entire process, including the unmyelinated tip and myelinated continuation, constitutes the peripheral process of a spiral ganglion (auditory) neuron. The spiral ganglion, as its name implies, lies within Rosenthal's canal that spirals from the base of the cochlea to its midpoint. At the midpoint, the canal disappears and ganglion cells become a confluent mass (see Figure 6–2). In contrast to other species, most human spiral ganglion cell bodies are unmyelinated.

Most (90–95%) of the spiral ganglion neurons are large round cells, 25 to 30 μm in diameter, whose peripheral processes contact the bases of inner hair cells. These larger neurons are designated type I ganglion cells, and they innervate inner hair cells in a highly convergent manner. Each inner hair cell in the midportion of the cochlea has synaptic junctions with the peripheral processes of as many as 15 spiral ganglion cells. Inner hair cells located toward the base or apex of the cochlea are contacted by a smaller number of processes, but it remains true that each inner hair cell drives a number of type I ganglion cells with its activity. A separate affer-

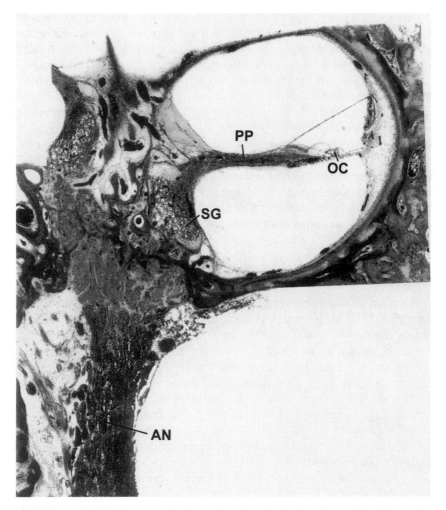

Figure 6–4. A microphotograph of a section through the human cochlea, illustrating the formation of the auditory nerve and its passage through the internal auditory canal. Iron hematoxylin stain. AN = auditory nerve; OC = organ of Corti; PP = peripheral processes; SG = spiral ganglion.

ent system is formed by the type II ganglion neurons, smaller neurons with a concentration of neurofilaments in their cytoplasm, which receive input from outer hair cells. Type II ganglion cells constitute only 5–10% of the total number of cells in the spiral ganglion, and their thin unmyelinated peripheral processes branch to synapse with a number of outer hair cells. The result of this organization is that the central processes of type I ganglion cells, carrying input from inner hair cells, constitute almost the entire volume of the afferent auditory nerve as it passes into the internal auditory canal within the temporal bone. Near the outlet from the internal auditory canal, the porus acusticus, there is an abrupt change in the myelin sheath from one produced by Schwann cells of the peripheral nervous system (Figure 6–5) to one produced by oligodendroglial cells of the central nervous system. It is this glial portion of the nerve that exits from the internal auditory canal to cross the intradural space.

The human auditory brain stem response (ABR) is known to be generated by the auditory nerve and brain stem structures, and its use as a diagnostic tool has prompted attempts to find the generators of individual ABR waves. Intrasurgical recordings, made with a wire electrode placed directly on the brain stem and auditory nerve (Moller & Jannetta, 1982), indicated that the first two ABR waves are generated before the entrance of the nerve into the brain stem. This interpretation was supported by clinical findings in a case of severe brain stem gliosis, in which ABR waves I and II were present, but all subsequent waves were absent (Kaga, Ono, Yokumaru, Owada, & Mizutani, 1998). In attempting to distinguish the

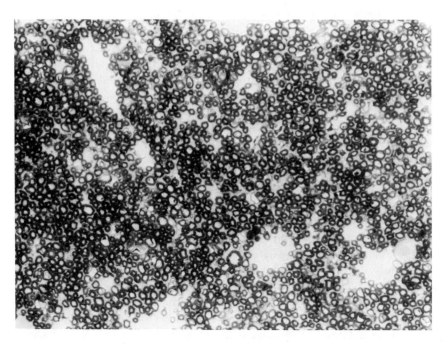

Figure 6–5. A high-power microphotograph of a cross-section through the human auditory nerve. Osmium-toluidin blue.

actual sites of generation of waves I and II, Buchwald (1983) summarized a body of evidence from animal studies suggesting that ABR wave I reflects a generator potential (i.e., graded activity in the terminal portion of the peripheral processes). This evidence includes the fact that wave I recorded from the scalp or middle-ear cavity is simultaneous with the first neural response recorded from the round window. In addition, sectioning of the nerve at the internal acoustic meatus leaves wave I intact but abolishes all subsequent ABR waves. It is generally assumed that wave I is generated by activation of the dendritic tips of afferent nerve fibers, in both man and other species.

In the case of ABR wave II, the situation in humans and animals differs because of the different lengths of the auditory nerve. In mammals such as the cat, the auditory nerve traverses only a few millimeters from the cochlea to the brain stem. In humans, the auditory nerve is 20–25 mm long because of the much larger cerebrospinal fluid compartment surrounding the human brain (see Figure 6–1). In recordings made during surgery (Martin, Pratt, & Schwegler, 1995), a potential corresponding to wave II of the scalp-recorded ABR was recorded from the nerve as it passed through the internal auditory meatus and crossed the intradural space. That study, as well as dipole localization studies (Scherg & von Cramon, 1985), concluded that human wave II is generated as the auditory nerve action potentials cross the conductivity boundaries at the interfaces of temporal bone, cerebrospinal fluid space, and brain stem.

The auditory nerve terminates shortly after it reaches the brain stem and enters the ventral cochlear nucleus. In recordings made from the human brain stem (Moller & Jannetta, 1982), a potential that coincided with wave III of the scalp-recorded ABR record was recorded on the brain stem surface just medial to the cochlear nuclei. The human dipole localization studies (Scherg & von Cramon, 1985) also placed wave III in or near the cochlear nuclei at the periphery of the brain stem. Based on this evidence, it is generally assumed that wave III is generated by action potentials in the axons leaving the cochlear nuclei and forming pathways to higher brain stem nuclei. If ABR wave III in fact represents the initial volley of action potentials in the brain stem, then subsequent ABR waves must be generated by these higher brain stem centers.

As mentioned previously, ABR recordings in subjects with auditory neuropathy are either highly distorted or completely absent, beginning with wave I. Because a recordable potential requires a synchronous volley of action potentials in a population of axons, the absence of waves I and II implies a lack of synchronous firing to transient stimuli in the auditory nerve from the point of synapse with the cochlear hair cells. The absence of waves III to VI does not necessarily imply pathology of central auditory nuclei, because if synchrony is lacking in the firing pattern of the auditory nerve, it will not be present in the brain stem pathways which relay the auditory nerve input. Still, there is presently no way to evaluate conduction in central pathways directly or to determine if conditions affecting conductivity in peripheral axons might also affect central axons.

CONCLUSIONS

The clinical observations in auditory neuropathy patients provide some clues to site of the pathologic process, if not its exact nature. The presence of the cochlear microphonic and of otoacoustic emissions in these patients seems to indicate that the pathology is not a loss of the outer hair cell motility system, either of its stereociliary or of its somatic components. In contrast, there is a general impairment of functions depending on neural elements. Activation of efferent axons does not produce normal suppression of otoacoustic emissions (see Hood and Berlin, Chapter 10 in this volume). The lack of an ABR suggests that transient stimuli do not produce synchronized firing in the afferent pathway. As pointed out by Starr et al. (1991), there is presently no adequate diagnostic procedure to evaluate the function of inner hair cells or the afferent synapse. To date, understanding the differential loss of function in auditory neuropathy has led to its diagnosis. Hopefully, with further investigations, these insights will lead to effective treatments.

REFERENCES

Berlin, C. I., Hood, L. J., Cecola, R. P., Jackson, D. F., & Szabo, P. (1993a). Does type I afferent neuron dysfunction reveal itself through lack of efferent suppression? *Hearing Research, 65,* 40–50.

Berlin, C. I., Hood, L. J., Wen, H., Szabo, P., Cecola, R. P., Rigby, P., & Jackson, D. F. (1993b). Contralateral suppression of non-linear click-evoked otoacoustic emissions. *Hearing Research, 71,* 1–11.

Brownell, W. E. (1984). Microscopic observation of cochlear hair cell motility. *Scanning Electron Microscopy,* Pt 3, 1401–1406.

Brownell, W. E. (1990). Outer hair cell electromotility and otoacoustic emissions. *Ear and Hearing, 11,* 82–92.

Brownell, W. E., Bader, C. R., Bertrand, D., & de Ribaupierre, Y. (1985). Evoked mechanical responses of isolated cochlear outer hair cells. *Science, 227,* 194–196.

Brundin, L., Flock, A., & Canlon, B. (1989). Sound-induced motility of isolated cochlear outer hair cells is frequency-specific. *Nature, 14,* 814–816.

Buchwald, J. S. (1983). Generators. In E. J. Moore (Ed.), *Bases of auditory brain-stem evoked responses* (pp. 157–195). New York: Grune & Stratton.

Dallos, P., & Cheatham, M. A. (1976). Production of cochlear potentials by inner and outer hair cells. *Journal of the Acoustical Society of America, 60*, 510–512.

Dallos, P., He, D. Z., Lin, X., Sziklai, I., Mehta, S., & Evans, B. N. (1997). Acetylcholine, outer hair cell electromotility and the cochlear amplifier. *Journal of Neuroscience, 17*, 2212–2226.

Denk, W., Holt, J. R., Shepherd, G. M., & Corey, D. P. (1995). Calcium imaging of single stereocilia in hair cells: Localization of transduction channels at both ends of tip links. *Neuron, 15*, 1311–1321.

Doyle, K. J., Sininger, Y., & Starr, A. (1998). Auditory neuropathy. *Laryngoscope, 108*, 1374–1377.

Evans, B. N., & Dallos, P. (1993). Stereocilia displacement induced somatic motility of cochlear outer hair cells. *Proceedings of the National Academy of Science, 90*, 8347–8351.

Flock, A., Bretscher, A., & Weber, K. (1982). Immunohistochemical localization of several cytoskeletal proteins in inner ear sensory and supporting cells. *Hearing Research, 7*, 75–89.

Flock, A., Cheung, H. C., Flock, B., & Utter, G. (1981). Three sets of actin filaments in sensory cells of the inner ear. Identification and functional orientation determined by gel electrophoresis, immunofluorescence and electron microscopy. *Journal of Neurocytology, 10*, 133–147.

Flock, A., Flock, B., & Ulfendahl, M. (1986). Mechanisms of movement in outer hair cells and a possible structural basis. *Archives of Otorhinolaryngology, 243*, 83–90.

Furness, D. N., & Hackney, C. M. (1985). Cross-links between stereocilia in the guinea pig cochlea. *Hearing Research, 18*, 177–188.

Hudspeth, A. J. (1989). Mechanoelectrical transduction by hair cells of the bullfrog's sacculus. *Progress in Brain Research, 80*, 129–135.

Ishi, T., Murakami, Y., & Ballogh, K. (1967). Acetylcholinesterase activity in the efferent nerve fibers of the human inner ear. *Annals of Otology and Laryngology, 76*, 115–123.

Kaga, K., Ono, M., Yokumaru, K., Owada, M., & Mizutani, T. (1998). Brainstem pathology of infantile Gaucher's disease with only wave I and II of auditory brainstem response. *Journal of Laryngology and Otology, 112*, 1069–1073.

Mammano, F., & Ashmore, J. F. (1993). Reverse transduction measured in the isolated cochlea by laser Michelson interferometry. *Nature, 365*, 838–841.

Martin, W. H., Pratt, H., & Schwegler, J. W. (1995). The origin of the human auditory brain-stem response wave II. *EEG and Clinical Electrophysiology, 96*, 357–370.

Moller, A. R., & Jannetta, P. J. (1982). Auditory evoked potentials recorded intracranially from the brainstem in man. *Experimental Neurology, 78*, 144–157.

Moore, J. K., & Osen, K. K. (1979). The cochlear nuclei in man. *American Journal of Anatomy, 154*, 393–418.

Moore, J. K., Simmons, D. D., & Guan, Y.-L. (1999). The human olivocochlear system: Organization and development. *Audiology and Neuro-Otology, 4*, 311–325.

Nadol, J. B., Jr. (1983a). Serial section reconstruction of the neural pole of hair cells in the human organ of Corti. I. Inner hair cells. *Laryngoscope, 93*, 599–614.

Nadol, J. B., Jr. (1983b). Serial section reconstruction of the neural pole of hair cells in the human organ of Corti. II. Outer hair cells. *Laryngoscope, 93*, 780–791.

Pickles, J. O., Comis, S. D., & Osborne, M. P. (1984). Cross-links between stereocilia in the guinea pig organ of Corti, and their possible relation to sensory transduction. *Hearing Research, 15,* 103–112.

Ryan, A., & Dallos, P. (1975). Effect of absence of cochlear outer hair cells on behavioral auditory threshold. *Nature, 25,* 44–46.

Scherg, M., von Cramon, D. (1985). A new interpretation of the generators of BAEP waves I-V: Results of spatio-temporal dipole modeling. *EEG and Clinical Neurophysiology, 62,* 290–299.

Schuknecht, H. F., Churchill, J. A., & Doran, R. (1959). The localization of acetylcholinesterase in the cochlea. *Archives of Otolaryngology, 69,* 149–157.

Sellick, P. M., & Russell, I. J. (1980). The responses of inner hair cells to basilar membrane velocity during low-frequency auditory stimulation in the guinea pig. *Hearing Research, 2,* 439–445.

Spoendlin, H. (1985). Anatomy of cochlear innervation. *American Journal of Otolaryngology, 6,* 453–467.

Starr, A., McPherson, D., Patterson, J., Don, M., Luxford, W., Shannon, R., Sininger, Y., Tonakawa, L., & Waring, M. (1991). Absence of both auditory evoked potentials and auditory percepts dependent on timing cues. *Brain, 114,* 1157–1180.

Starr, A., Picton, T. W., Sininger, Y., Hood, L. J., & Berlin, C. I. (1996). Auditory neuropathy. *Brain, 119,* 741–753.

Sziklai, I., He, D. Z., & Dallos, P. (1996). Effect of acetylcholine and GABA on the transfer function of electromotility in isolated outer hair cells. *Hearing Research, 95,* 87–99.

Takasaka, T., Shirikawa, H., Hashimoto, S., Watanuki, K., & Kawamoto, K. (1983). High-voltage electron miroscopic study of the inner ear. *Annals of Otology, Rhinology and Laryngology, 92*(Suppl. 102), 1–12.

Wright, A. (1981). Scanning electron microscopy of the human cochlea—The organ of Corti. *Archives of Oto-Rhino-Laryngology, 230,* 11–19.

Zheng, J., Shen, W., He, D. Z., Long, K. B., Madison, L. D., & Dallos, P. (2000). Prestin is the motor protein of cochlear outer hair cells. *Nature, 405*(6783), 149–155.

Primary Cochlear Neuronal Degeneration

Joseph B. Nadol, Jr.

Degeneration of the spiral ganglion cell and its processes may occur as a secondary or as a primary event (Zimmermann, Nadol, & Burgess, 1995). Secondary cochlear neuronal degeneration is thought to follow a variety of insults to the organ of Corti. Primary cochlear neuronal degeneration, both in humans and in animals, has been described in a variety of pathologies, including genetic, toxic, metabolic, immune-mediated, degenerative, idiopathic, and infectious disorders. Degeneration of the inner ear rarely affects a single target tissue, such as neurons. More often degeneration of a variety of structures occurs, and hence, it is often difficult to differentiate cochlear neuronal degeneration that is secondary to injury to the organ of Corti from primary cochlear neuronal degeneration. It is the purpose of this chapter to review the range of human diseases resulting in sensorineural loss in which there is a reasonable clinical suspicion, pathologic evidence, or both of predominant or primary cochlear neuronal degeneration (Table 7–1).

GENETICALLY INDUCED SENSORINEURAL LOSS

Peripheral Neuropathies and Hearing Loss

There are several reports of hereditary peripheral neuropathy associated with sensorineural hearing loss (Begeer, Scholte, & vanEssen, 1991; Hagemoser et al. 1989; Hanft & Haddad, 1994; Wright & Dyck, 1995). Audiometric studies have suggested neural dysfunction as a primary etiology of sensorineural loss in these disorders (Pareyson, Scaioli, Berta, & Sghirlanzoni, 1995; Satya-Murti, Cacace, & Hanson, 1979; Starr, Picton, Sininger,

Table 7–1. Putative etiologies of primary cochlear neuronal degeneration.

Genetic
Peripheral neuropathies and hearing loss
    Friedreich's ataxia
    Charcot-Marie-Tooth disease
    Usher's syndrome
    Refsum's disease
Mitochondrial genetic diseases (?)
DFN-1 (Mohr-Tranebjaerg syndrome)

Toxic or Metabolic
Diabetes mellitus (?)
Organic mercury poisoning
Uremia
Alcoholic neuropathy (?)
Hyperbilirubinemia

Immunologic
Polyarteritis nodosa
Cogan's syndrome
Lupus erythematosus
Multiple sclerosis

Degenerative
Neuronal presbycusis

Idiopathic
Sudden idiopathic sensorineural hearing loss
Meniere's syndrome
Paraneoplastic neuropathy

Infectious
Fungal meningitis
Herpes zoster oticus
Cytomegalic inclusion disease

Hood, & Berlin, 1996). Specific disease entities, in which peripheral neuropathy and sensorineural loss are predominant symptoms, include Friedreich's ataxia, Charcot-Marie-Tooth disease, Usher's syndrome, and Refsum's disease.

In Friedreich's ataxia, the evidence for primary neural dysfunction as a cause of sensorineural loss is based on behavioral audiometry and auditory evoked response testing. Thus, Quine, Regan, and Murray (1984) demonstrated abnormalities in response to pitch cues in speech-like sound. Amantini et al. (1984) and Ell, Prasher, and Rudge (1984) demonstrated evidence of brain stem dysfunction by auditory evoked response testing, and Taylor, McMenamin, Andermann, and Waters (1982) demonstrated abnormalities suggesting both cortical and peripheral neural dysfunction as a cause of sensorineural hearing loss. Likewise, Satya-Murti, Cacace, and Hanson (1980) and Shanon, Himelfarb, and Gold (1981) demonstrated abnormalities in behavioral audiometry and auditory evoked response testing consistent with the hypothesis that both the cochlear nerve and brain stem were the likely sites of pathology.

The only published histopathology of the inner ear in Friedreich's ataxia was presented by Spoendlin (1974). In two cases, the predominant histopathology was severe loss of cochlear neurons and spiral ganglion cells, increasing from base to apex, whereas the organ of Corti appeared to be essentially normal throughout the cochlea. Likewise, in the vestibular labyrinth, there was selective loss of neural elements.

In Charcot-Marie-Tooth disease, the evidence of primary cochlear neuronal dysfunction as causative for sensorineural loss, includes behavioral audiometry, auditory brain stem response (ABR), and electrocochleography, suggesting either primary 8th nerve dysfunction (Raglan, Prasher, Trinder, & Rudge, 1987) or, perhaps, central dysfunction (Musiek, Weider, & Mueller, 1982).

The molecular genetics of Charcot-Marie-Tooth disease seems to include several distinct abnormalities, the most common being abnormalities of peripheral myelin protein 22 (PMP–22) on chromosome 17p 11.2 (Chance & Fishbeck, 1994; Ouvrier 1996; Yoshikawa et al., 1994).

Similarly, the published pathology of the peripheral nerve in Charcot-Marie-Tooth disease seems to be variable and includes (a) primary neuronal atrophy, (b) a peripheral demyelinating process resulting in hypertrophic neuropathy and, finally, (c) a myopathy, with no obvious neuronal loss. Hypertrophic neuropathy in this disease has been described by Smith, Bhawan, Keller, and DeGirolami (1980) to include segmental demyelinization, remyelinization, axonal degeneration, and Schwann cell proliferation, quite similar to Djerine-Sottas disease.

Temporal bone histopathology is available in Charcot-Marie-Tooth syndrome (Figure 7–1). In this case, the primary lesion appears to be loss of cochlear spiral ganglion cells and hypertrophic change in cranial nerves VII and VIII.

Usher's syndrome is a genetically heterogeneous group of diseases. The disorder has been divided into three groups: 85% fall into group 1, characterized by profound congenital deafness, gait disturbance, and retinitis pigmentosa with onset before puberty; 10% of patients fall into group 2, which is characterized by severe congenital deafness, rare gait disturbances, and retinitis pigmentosa with onset after puberty; and, finally, 5% of patients fall into group 3, characterized by a progressive sensorineural hearing loss with retinitis pigmentosa.

Temporal bone histopathology is available both at a light and electron microscope level (Figures 7–2, 7–3, and 7–4). In both cases reported from our laboratory (Belal 1975; Shinkawa & Nadol, 1986), there was

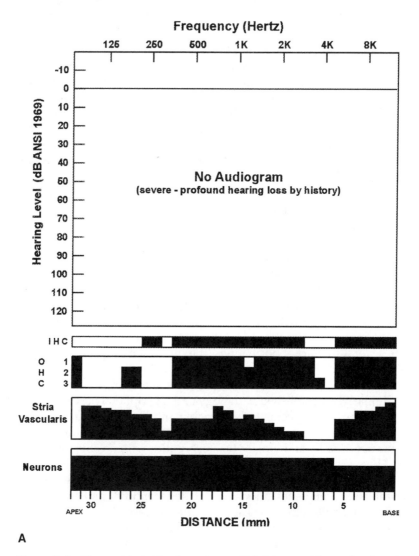

A

Figure 7–1. Charcot-Marie-Tooth syndrome. This 74-year-old man developed progressive peripheral neuropathies beginning in midlife. At approximately 50 years of age, he developed a slowly progressive bilateral sensorineural loss, and by history he was severely deaf in both ears 3 years prior to death at age 74. Neurologic evaluation confirmed the diagnosis of Charcot-Marie-Tooth syndrome. **A.** Cytocochleogram of the left temporal bone. There was severe loss of neurons throughout the cochlea. In addition, there was patchy atrophy of the stria vascularis and of inner and outer hair cells. **B.** Midmodiolar section through the left temporal bone. There was severe loss of spiral ganglion cells (SPG) in all turns of the cochlea. H & E stain. Mag. = 25×. **C.** Despite severe loss of spiral ganglion cells, there appeared to be a hypertrophic neuropathy of nerves within the internal auditory canal, including cranial nerves VII and VIII. Luxol Fast Blue/cresyl violet strain. Mag. = 14.5×.

102

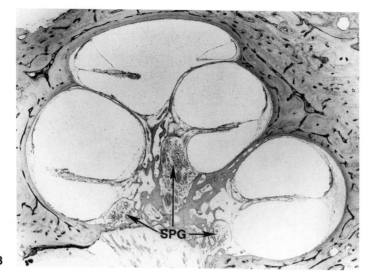

B

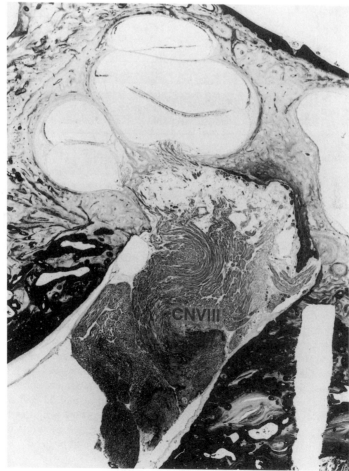

C

103

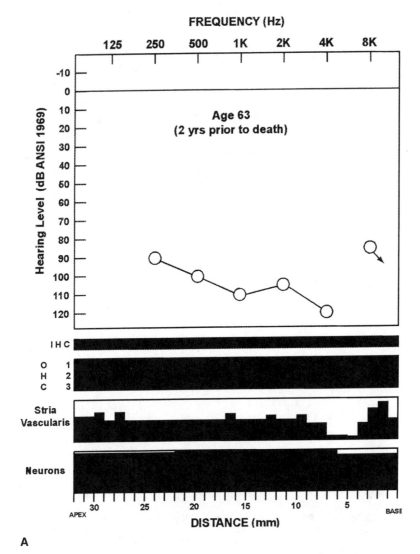

FREQUENCY (Hz)

Age 63
(2 yrs prior to death)

A

Figure 7–2. Usher's syndrome type I. A 65-year-old man was profoundly deaf, presumably from birth. There was progressive loss of vision starting in the second decade of life, diagnosed as retinitis pigmentosa. **A.** Cytocochleogram of right ear. Audiometry 2 years before death demonstrated severe-to-profound sensorineural loss. There was total loss of inner and outer hair cells and almost complete loss of spiral ganglion cells. In addition, there was atrophy of the stria vascularis. **B.** Midmodiolar section of the right temporal bone. Almost no spiral ganglion cells were visible within Rosenthal's canal. H & E stain. Mag. = 26×. **C.** Basal turn of the right temporal bone. There is almost total absence of spiral ganglion cells in Rosenthal's canal (R). No neurons were visible within the osseous spiral lamina (OSL). There was complete atrophy of the organ of Corti (OC). H & E stain. Mag. = 54×.

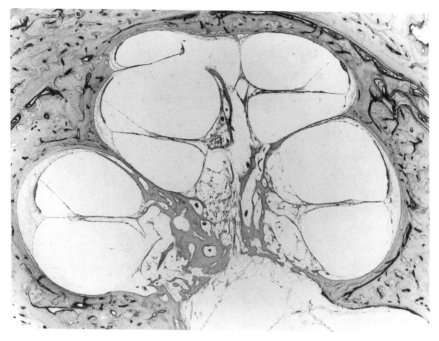

B

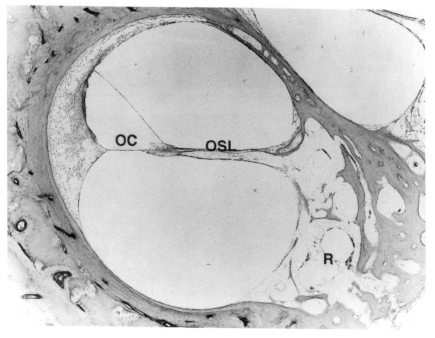

C

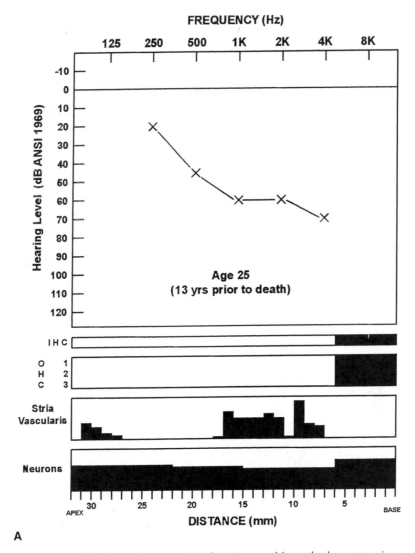

A

Figure 7–3. Usher's syndrome type III. This 38-year-old man had a progressive sensorineural loss beginning in childhood. At age 25, ophthalmologic examination confirmed a diagnosis of retinitis pigmentosa. **A.** Cytocochleogram of the left ear. There was moderate-to-severe loss of spiral ganglion cells in all turns of the cochlea. There was patchy atrophy of the stria vascularis. The organ of Corti was normal with the exception of loss of hair cells in the basal 6 mm. **B.** Midmodiolar section of the left temporal bone. There was loss of spiral ganglion cells, particularly in the basal turn. H & E stain. Mag. = 28×. **C.** Organ of Corti in the basal turn of the left temporal bone. Although both inner and outer hair cells were present, there was marked loss of neurons within the osseous spiral lamina (OSL). H & E stain. Mag. = 195×.

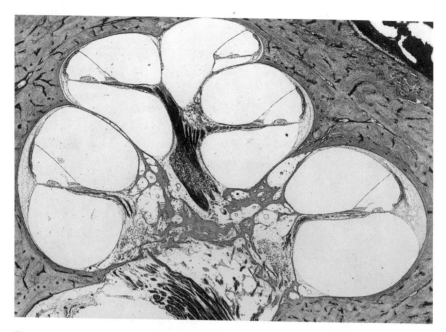

B

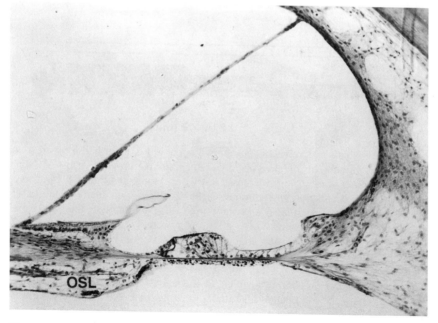

OSL

C

107

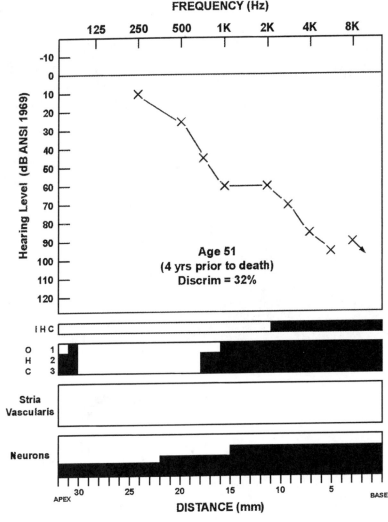

A

Figure 7–4. Usher's syndrome type III. This 55-year-old woman had a progressive bilateral sensorineural hearing loss beginning in childhood. Progressive loss of vision led to a diagnosis of retinitis pigmentosa. **A.** Cytocochleogram of the left ear. There was loss of spiral ganglion cells throughout the cochlea, particularly in the basal turn. There was also loss of inner and outer hair cells, particularly in the basal turn. Speech discrimination score was 32% in both ears, consistent with neural dysfunction. **B.** Midmodiolar section through the left temporal bone. There was marked loss of spiral ganglion cells in the basal turn. H & E stain. Mag. = 24×. **C.** Basal turn in the left temporal bone. Despite a normal-appearing organ of Corti (OC), there was marked loss of spiral ganglion cells (SPG). H & E stain. Mag. = 64.2×. **D.** Electron micrograph of an abnormal radial fiber under the inner hair cell in the basal turn of the right ear. Although the fiber was of normal caliber as it passed through the basilar membrane, under the inner hair cell it expanded into a large club-like process approximately 15 μm in diameter and contained whirls of neurofilament (NF) and myelin figures (MF). Mag. = 5,500×.

108

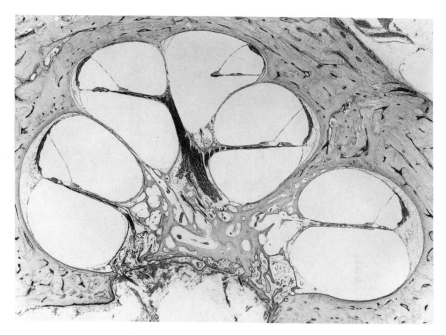

B

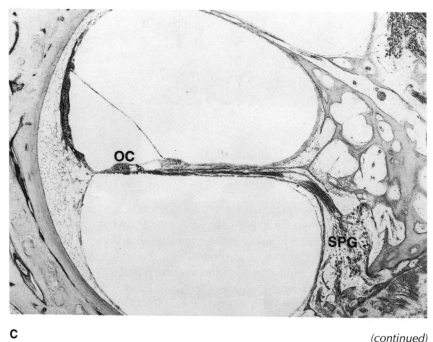

C

(continued)

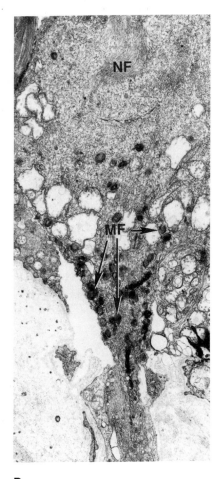

D

Figure 7–4. *(continued)*

loss of elements of the organ of Corti and neuronal loss. In the case for which electron microscopy was available, however, behavioral audiometry strongly suggested a primary cochlear neuronal degeneration because of the sharply down sloping sensorineural loss and poor speech discrimination. Cochlear neuronal degeneration was seen both by light and electron microscopy. Ultrastructural evidence of neuronal degeneration included pathologic changes in the spiral ganglion, peripheral dendrites, and a decrease in the number of afferent endings at the base of both inner and outer hair cells (Nadol 1988a, 1988b).

Refsum's Disease

Refsum's disease is an autosomal recessive disorder characterized by polyneuritis, cerebellar ataxia, atypical retinitis pigmentosa, peripheral neuropathy, cataracts, congenital icthyosis, cardiac myopathy, and sensorineural hearing loss. An elevated serum phythanic acid is characteristic. Pathology of the peripheral neuron includes hypertrophic neuropathy involving a demyelinization and remyelinization phenomenon.

Temporal bone histopathology is available in Refsum's disease. Again, the primary lesion within the inner ear appears to be degeneration of the first order cochlear neuron (Figure 7–5).

MITOCHONDRIAL GENETIC DISEASES

There are at least three varieties of mitochondrial disease, including (a) Kearns-Sayre syndrome, characterized by pigment degeneration in the retina, external ophthalmoplegia, other cranial neuropathies, complete heart block, and sensorineural hearing loss; (b) MELAS syndrome (mitochondrial encephalopathy, lactic acidosis, and stroke-like episodes); and (c) MERRF syndrome (myoclonus, epilepsy, and ragged red muscle fibers). In Kearns-Sayre syndrome, the most common genetic lesion is a 4977 base pair deletion of mitochondrial DNA in position 8482 to 13,459. In the MELAS syndrome, the most common genetic abnormality is a point mutation (A to G) at position 3243 in mitochondrial transfer RNA. This point mutation is also seen in diabetes and sensorineural hearing loss without full-blown MELAS syndrome. In the MELAS syndrome, several clinical symptoms would suggest primary neural dysfunction, including transient cortical blindness, hemianopsia, focal paresis, paralysis, and dysphagia. Audiometric studies of hearing loss (which is common, if not universal in this syndrome) have demonstrated flat sensorineural hearing loss with excellent speech discrimination, however, suggestive of cochlear dysfunction (Donovan, 1995; Oshima, Ueda, Ikeda, Abe, & Takasaka, 1996). Similarly, ABR and evoked otoacoustic emissions also suggest cochlear rather than neuronal lesion (Yamasoba, Oka, Tsukuda, Nakamura, & Kaga, 1996). Nevertheless, the audiometric studies of Elverland and Torbergsen (1991) suggested that the early lesion is consistent with cochlear dysfunction, whereas the late lesion in this study included evidence of retrocochlear or neuronal dysfunction. Histopathology is available in the Kearns-Sayre syndrome (Lindsay & Hinojosa, 1976). Although there was degeneration of the organ of Corti and stria vascularis, there also was marked degeneration of the spiral ganglion cells.

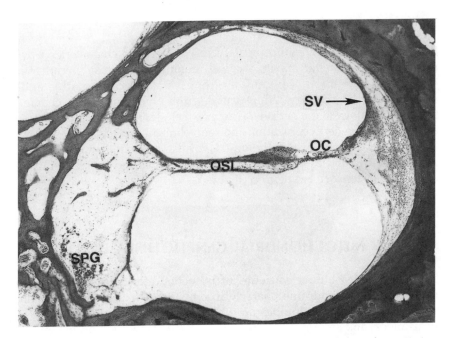

Figure 7–5. Refsum's disease. This 38-year-old man developed a bilateral progressive sensorineural loss starting approximately at age 17. Visual impairment had been present since childhood. Weakness of the lower extremities began at approximately age 15. Neurologic evaluation revealed severe diffuse peripheral neuropathies, and a diagnosis of Refsum's disease was made by a neurologic consultant. Photomicrograph of the organ of Corti and spiral ganglion in the basal turn of the left temporal bone. There was collapse of Reissner's membrane against an atrophied stria vascularis (SV) and organ of Corti (OC). There was marked loss of spiral ganglion cells (SPG) in Rosenthal's canal and no dendritic fibers visible within the osseous spiral lamina (OSL). H & E stain. Mag. = 65.2×.

Another genetic disorder that relates to mitochondrial function is the Mohr-Tranebjaerg syndrome (DFN–1). First described as a nonsyndromic x-linked disorder mapped to Xq22, it is now known that affected individuals also demonstrate dystonia, mental deficiency, and blindness (Jin et al., 1996). The cloned gene encodes the "deafness/dystonia peptide," (DDP), which is a nuclear encoded mitochondrial transport protein. A mutation in this protein causes defective transport of metabolites from the cytoplasm to the mitochondrial inner membrane and hence defective oxidative phosphorylation (Koehler et al., 1999).

The most striking histopathologic change is near total atrophy of the cochlear neurons and preservation of the organ of Corti (Figure 7–6).

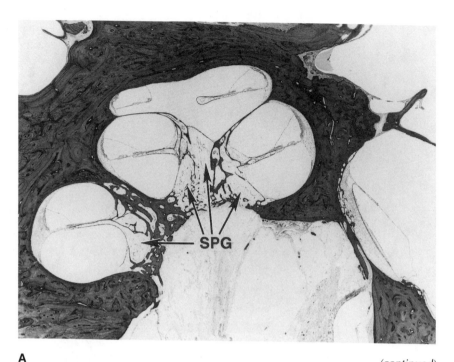

A

(continued)

Figure 7–6. Mohr-Tranebjaerg syndrome (DFN–1). This 67-year-old man was deaf at least since the age of 4 years. He became blind at age 58 years after 10 years of failing vision. Dystonia and dysphagia were noted at age 57. **A.** Midmodiolar section of right temporal bone shows near total loss (9% remaining of mean normal for age) of spiral ganglion cells (SPG). H & E stain. Mag. = 17.4×. **B.** Photomicrograph of basal turn of the cochlea. The organ of Corti (OC) was intact, whereas there was nearly total loss of spiral ganglion cells (SPG). H & E stain. Mag. = 62.5×.

TOXIC OR METABOLIC CAUSES OF PRIMARY COCHLEAR NEURONAL DEGENERATION

Diabetes Mellitus

A variety of manifestations of neural dysfunction has been described in association with diabetes mellitus. In a study of hearing loss in diabetics with peripheral neuropathy, regression analysis demonstrated a significantly higher hearing threshold in the diabetic group as compared to age-matched control subjects, suggesting neuropathy of the auditory nerve (Friedman, Schulman, & Weiss, 1975). Similarly, elevation of pure-tone auditory thresholds in diabetic patients was described by Ferrer et al.

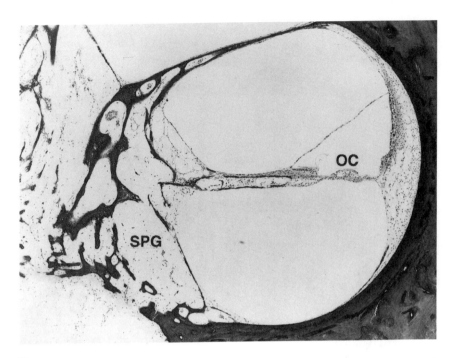

B

Figure 7–6. *(continued)*

(1991). In addition, significant associations between auditory threshold elevation, age, duration of disease, and diabetic retinopathy, but not with diabetic neuropathy, were shown. Other studies (Harner, 1981), however, failed to show any association of diabetes with hearing loss as compared to age-matched control subjects. At the present time, the clinical and histopathologic evidence, based on temporal bone studies (Schuknecht, 1993) would suggest little or no effect of diabetes on the peripheral hearing organ and, despite other cranial and peripheral neuropathies, no direct evidence of effect on the cochlear neuron.

Organic Mercury Poisoning

Significant neurologic dysfunction has been demonstrated in organic mercury poisoning (chronic Minimata disease). This includes sensory impairment in the extremities, alteration of visual fields, retrocochlear hearing loss, and cerebellar incoordination (Uchino et al., 1995). In experimental poisoning in rats, both cutaneous and auditory dysfunction have been demonstrated (Wu, Ison, Wecker, & Lapham, 1985). Although peripheral or central auditory neuronal dysfunction is suspected in this disorder, to date no temporal bone histopathology is available.

Uremia

The clinical neuropathologic changes associated with renal failure including hearing loss are well known. A case study of one such patient demonstrated cochlear as well as neuronal dysfunction (Anteunis & Mooy, 1987). Abnormalities including conduction velocity in the uremic state were reversible following renal transplantation, suggesting an auditory neuronal dysfunction as a possibility in at least some uremic patients.

Alcoholic Neuropathy

The peripheral polyneuropathy associated with chronic alcoholism is well known. To date, however, no convincing control studies have demonstrated any significant physiologic or histologic evidence of damage to the inner ear.

It is likely that a variety of chemicals may have ototoxic effects, possibly including primary effects on the cochlear neuron (Rybak, 1992; Spitzer, 1981)

Hyperbilirubinemia

Hearing loss has been described in severe neonatal hyperbilirubinemia. The audiometric pattern consists of a downsloping sensorineural loss with decreased speech discrimination. A retrocochlear site of lesion, either the auditory nerve or brain stem, has been suggested by human auditory evoked responses (Chisin, Perlman, & Sohner, 1979; Nwaesei, VanAerde, Boyden, & Perlman, 1984; Perlman et al. 1983) and findings in the jaundiced Gunn rat (Shapiro, & Hecox, 1989; Uziel, Marot, & Pujol, 1983). Concomitant neurologic manifestations, including encephalopathy, extrapyramidal signs, chorioathetosis, and seizures would also suggest significant neural dysfunction in addition to hearing loss. The only histopathology that is available on the auditory pathway in human hyperbilirubinemia is cited by Goodhill (1967). In three human temporal bone specimens, the organ of Corti appeared normal, but there was some degeneration of the spiral ganglion. More central auditory structures were not examined, however. The best clinical evidence to date suggests that hyperbilirubinemia causes hearing loss by involvement of central neural pathways and, perhaps, the 8th cranial nerve.

SYSTEMIC IMMUNE DISORDERS

Neurologic abnormalities and sensorineural hearing loss are prominent symptoms in a variety of systemic immune-mediated disorders, including polyarteritis nodosa, Cogan's syndrome, and lupus erythematosus. Although primary involvement of the auditory nerve might be suspected on the basis of neuropathy in other parts of the body, available histopathology of the temporal bone in systemic immune disorders suggest degeneration of the organ of Corti and stria vascularis, new bone formation within the ear, and endolymphatic hydrops (Schuknecht & Nadol, 1994), perhaps reflecting a common pathogenesis consisting of ischemia secondary to vasculitis rather than a primary immunologic attack on neuronal structures.

Multiple Sclerosis

Despite the other predominant neurologic symptoms, no consistent pattern of hearing loss has been documented, although retrocochlear involvement has been described (Citron, Dix, Hallpike, & Hood, 1963). Auditory evoked response testing also has suggested involvement of the auditory pathways in the brain stem (Hausler & Levine, 1980). Direct involvement of the distal auditory nerve has been suggested by Bergamaschi (Bergamaschi, Romani, Zapoli, Versino, & Cosi, 1997). It is probable that multiple sclerosis may involve the auditory pathway from the auditory nerve throughout the brain stem and midbrain (Maurer, Schafer, Hopf, & Leitner, 1980). Histopathology of the auditory pathways is not available.

AGING AND DEGENERATIVE DISORDERS

Schuknecht has described five common varieties of presbycusis, which include primary degeneration of cochlear hair cells, primary degeneration of the stria vascularis, primary degeneration of cochlear neurons, and an indeterminate group (Schuknecht, 1964). Although pure cochlear neuronal degeneration is rarely seen in human presbycusis, there nevertheless are clearly cases in which the predominant histopathologic correlate of hearing loss in this disorder is loss of the spiral ganglion cell and its processes (Figures 7–7 and 7–8). Ultrastructural studies of such cases have also demonstrated degenerative changes in spiral ganglion cells, peripheral processes, and afferent synapses (Nadol, 1979; Nadol, 1988b) (Figure 7–9).

In the neural subtype of presbycusis as well as other varieties, it is not clear if the pathogenesis is true aging or whether it represents a

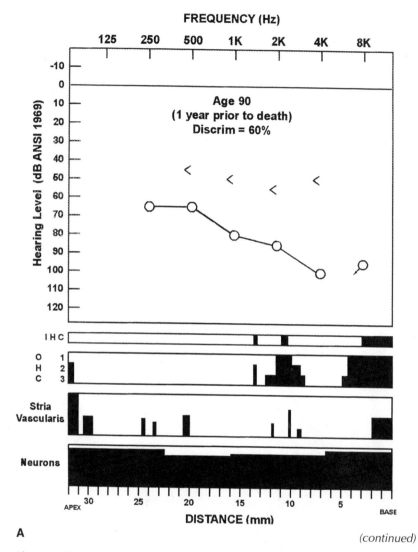

A

(continued)

Figure 7–7. Neural presbycusis. This 91-year-old woman had a history of slowly progressive bilateral sensorineural loss for more than 10 years. Audiometry revealed bilateral sensorineural loss with a downsloping pattern and reduced speech discrimination score consistent with neural presbycusis. **A.** Cytocochleogram of the right temporal bone. The principal histopathologic correlate of hearing loss was severe loss of cochlear neurons throughout the cochlea. **B.** Midmodiolar section through the right temporal bone. There was severe loss of spiral ganglion cells in all turns of the cochlea despite preservation of the organ of Corti. H & E stain. Mag. = 28×. **C.** Photomicrograph of the basal turn of the cochlea. The organ of Corti (OC) appeared normal. There was severe loss of spiral ganglion cells (SPG) and dendritic fibers in the osseous spiral lamina (OSL). H & E stain. Mag. = 66×.

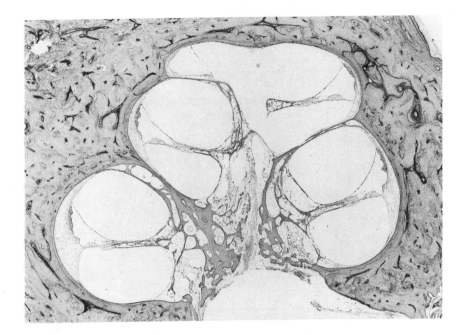

B

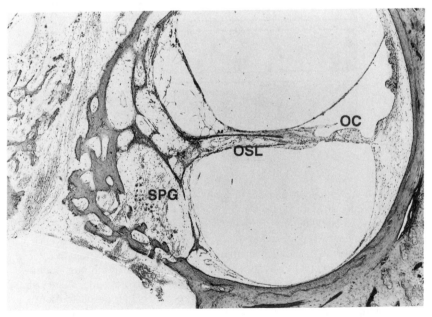

C

Figure 7–7. *(continued)*

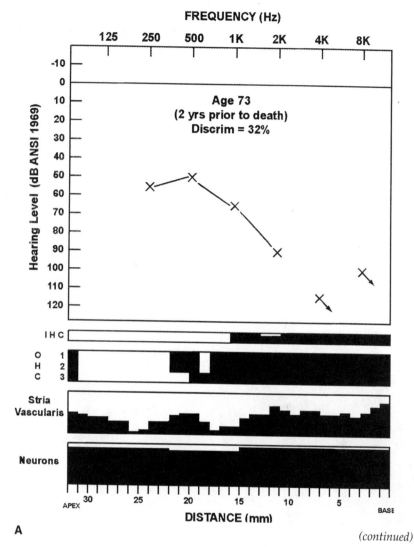

A

(continued)

Figure 7–8. Neural presbycusis. This 74-year-old man developed progressive bilateral symmetrical sensorineural loss starting at the age of 57. Two years before death, audiometry demonstrated bilateral downsloping sensorineural loss with reduced speech discrimination. **A.** Cytocochleogram of the left ear. The predominant histopathologic correlate of the hearing loss was loss of spiral ganglion cells throughout the cochlea and loss of inner and outer hair cells, particularly in basal half of the cochlea. **B.** Midmodiolar section through the left temporal bone. There was marked loss of spiral ganglion cells, particularly in the basal turn. H & E stain. Mag. = 25×. **C.** Photomicrograph of Rosenthal's canal of the basal turn. Only a few spiral ganglion cells (SPG) remained in Rosenthal's canal. H & E stain. Mag. = 105×.

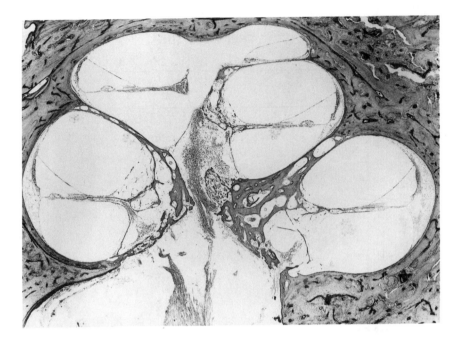

B

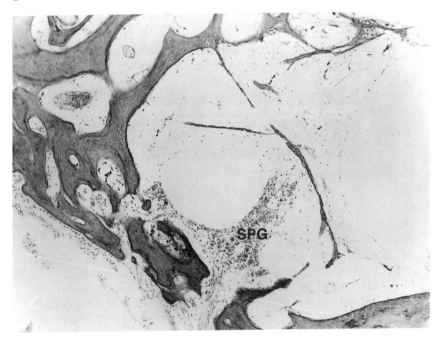

C

Figure 7–8. *(continued)*

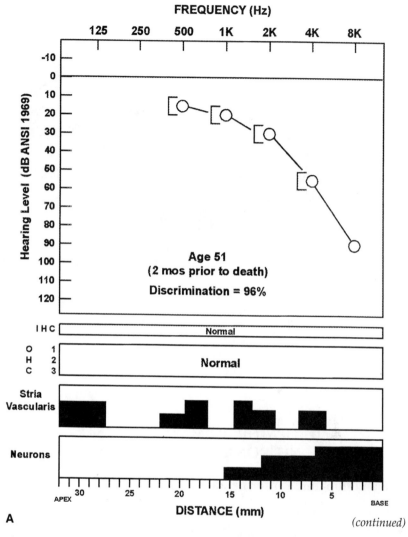

FREQUENCY (Hz)

Age 51
(2 mos prior to death)
Discrimination = 96%

IHC — Normal

OHC 1 2 3 — Normal

Stria Vascularis

Neurons

APEX 30 25 20 15 10 5 BASE

DISTANCE (mm)

A

(continued)

Figure 7–9. Neural presbycusis. This 51-year-old man had a progressive hearing loss in his right ear for many years. There had been a total loss of hearing in the left ear of unknown cause for at least 30 years. Audiometry 2 months before death showed a downsloping audiometric pattern with speech discrimination of 96%. **A.** Cytocochleogram of the right temporal bone. The principal histopathologic correlate of the sensorineural loss was loss of spiral ganglion cells in the basal turn. **B.** Transmission electron micrograph of dendritic fibers in the basal turn at 8 mm from the round window. There was disorganization of the myelin sheaths and myelin figures (MF) within the cytoplasm of surrounding schwann cells. Mag. = 7,500×.

121

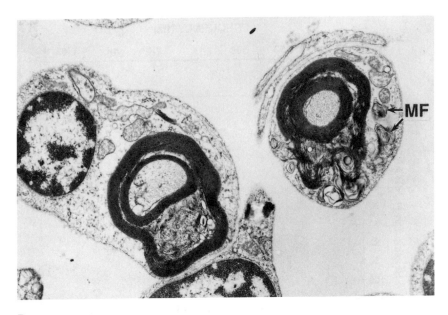

B

Figure 7–9. *(continued)*

yet undiagnosed genetically determined progressive neural degeneration in the inner ear.

IDIOPATHIC PRIMARY COCHLEAR NEURONAL DEGENERATION

Sudden Idiopathic Sensorineural Loss

Although the most common histopathologic correlate of sudden idiopathic sensorineural hearing loss is a generalized loss of both cochlear and neuronal structures within the inner ear, there have been examples in which the primary target appeared to be the cochlear neuron itself (Ishii & Toriyama, 1977; Schuknecht & Donovan, 1986) (Figures 7–10 and 7–11).

Ménière's Syndrome

The characteristic audiometric changes in Ménière's syndrome include, in addition to other findings, a progressive loss of speech discrimination (Enander & Stahle, 1967; Holmgren, 1964; Meurman & Grahne, 1956; Stahle, 1976), suggesting neural dysfunction. The primary histopathologic

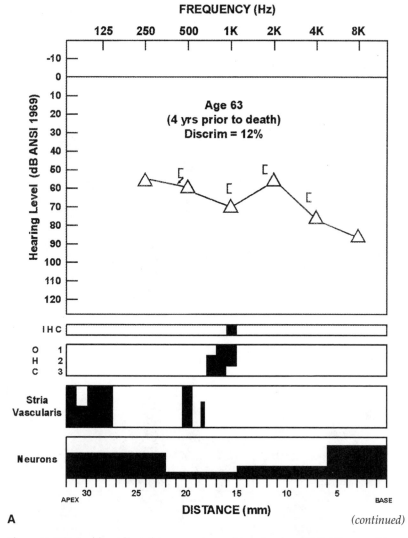

A

(continued)

Figure 7–10. Sudden idiopathic sensorineural hearing loss. This 67-year-old man developed a sudden loss of hearing in his right ear at age 63. This was accompanied by mild vertigo. Audiometry at that time demonstrated down-sloping sensorineural loss with markedly reduced speech discrimination (12%). **A.** Cytocochleogram of the right ear. There was loss of spiral ganglion cells throughout the cochlea. In addition, there was moderate loss of hair cells and patchy atrophy of the stria vascularis. **B.** Midmodiolar section of the right temporal bone. There was loss of spiral ganglion cells throughout the cochlea. H & E stain. Mag. = 25.6×. **C.** Despite loss of spiral ganglion cells, the organ of Corti, including inner (IHC), and outer hair cells (OHC), were still present in the basal turn. H & E stain. Mag. = 460×.

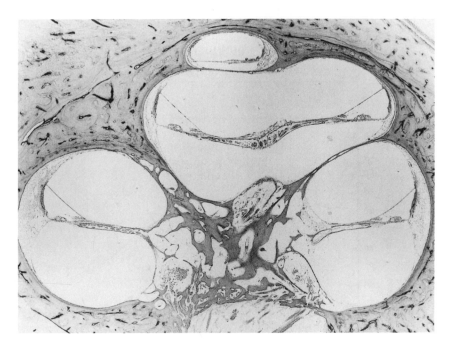

B

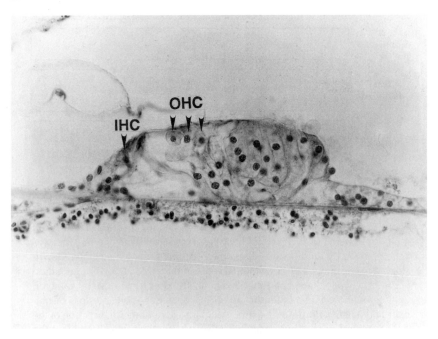

C

Figure 7–10. *(continued)*

124

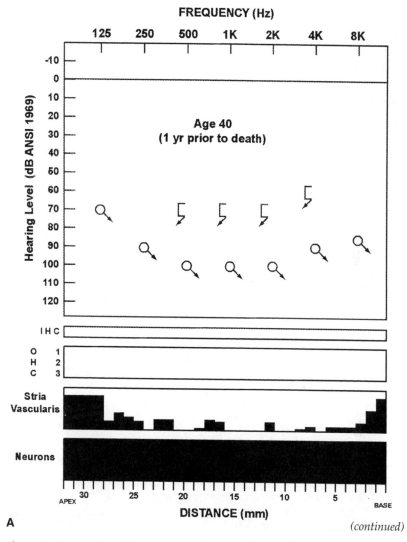

FREQUENCY (Hz)

A

(continued)

Figure 7–11. Sudden idiopathic sensorineural hearing loss. This 41-year-old man developed a sudden loss of hearing in the right ear at age 18. Profound sensorineural loss was documented by audiometry 1 year before death. **A.** Cytocochleogram of the right ear. There was a total loss of spiral ganglion cells throughout the cochlea despite good preservation of inner and outer hair cells. **B.** Photomicrograph of the basal turn of the cochlea. Rosenthal's canal (R) was totally devoid of spiral ganglion cells. H & E stain. Mag. = 52×. **C.** Organ of Corti of the basal turn. Despite some compression artifact, both inner (IHC) and outer (OHC) hair cells were visible. H & E stain. Mag. = 450×.

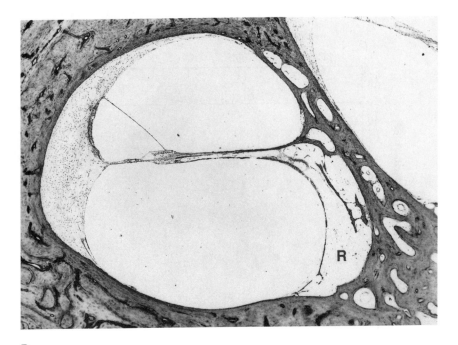

B

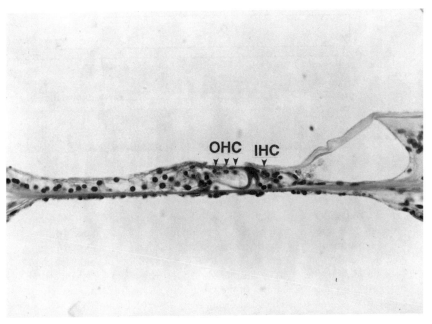

C

Figure 7–11. *(continued)*

126

correlate of Ménière's syndrome includes endolymphatic hydrops (Schuknecht, Benitez, & Beekhuis, 1962) and loss of cochlear hair cells and neurons, particularly in the apical turn. It has been repeatedly demonstrated that the degree of loss of hair cells and neurons does not correlate with the severity of hearing loss, however, particularly in advanced cases (Lindsay, Kohut, & Sciarra, 1967; Schuknecht, 1975; Schuknecht et al., 1962; Figure 7–12). In a case of unilateral Ménière's syndrome studied by electron microscopy (Nadol & Thornton, 1987), a significant decrease in the number of afferent nerve endings and afferent synapses at the base of both inner and outer hair cells was detected. The predominant location of pathology seemed to be the dendritic arborization of the spiral ganglion cell, which was undetectable by light microscopy. Similar changes can be seen in experimental hydrops in the guinea pig (Nadol, Adams, & Kim, 1995; Figure 7–13). In the experimental animal, electrophysiologic studies have demonstrated marked decrement in cochlear frequency selectivity, in addition to threshold elevation (Harrison, 1988), alterations in single cochlear neuron responses (Harrison & Prijs, 1984), and reduction in sensitivity and frequency selectivity of primary cochlear nerve responses (Lounsbury-Martin, Martin, Coats, & Johnson, 1988), all suggestive of primary dysfunction of the cochlear neuron.

Paraneoplastic Neuropathy

Some malignancies, particularly oat cell carcinoma of the lung and carcinoma of the stomach and ovary, may produce neurologic symptoms by mechanisms other than direct tumor invasion (Figure 7–14). Sensory and motor neurons may be affected. The pathophysiology of neural dysfunction is unknown but thought to be either immune-mediated or perhaps a form of dysmetabolic neuropathy.

INFECTIONS OF THE INNER EAR

Fungal Meningitis

In hearing loss caused by fungal meningitis, audiometric evidence suggested involvement of both the cochlea and the auditory nerve (Nadol, 1978). Temporal bone histopathology in cryptococcal meningitis has demonstrated a predilection for neural involvement by fungal granulomas within the inner ear (Igarashi, Weber, Alford, Coats, & Jerger, 1975; McGill, 1978; Figure 7–15).

Herpes Zoster Oticus (Ramsay Hunt Syndrome)

This disorder, caused by the neurotropic varicella-zoster virus, produces cutaneous pain secondary to involvement of sensory nerves, as well as

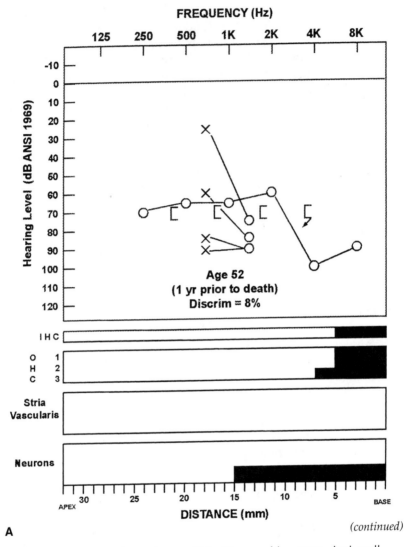

FREQUENCY (Hz)

Age 52
(1 yr prior to death)
Discrim = 8%

IHC

O 1
H 2
C 3

Stria
Vascularis

Neurons

APEX   30   25   20   15   10   5   BASE

DISTANCE (mm)

A

(continued)

Figure 7–12. Ménière's syndrome. This 53-year-old woman had well-documented right Ménière's syndrome starting at age 52 with right-sided tinnitus, hearing loss, dizziness, and reduced vestibular response on the right. **A.** Cytocochleogram of the right ear. Despite a moderate-to-severe sensorineural loss with markedly reduced speech discrimination, there was only modest loss of neurons in the basal turn and hair cells, and both inner (IHC) and outer (OHC) were present except in the basal 5–7 mm. **B.** Midmodiolar section of the right temporal bone. There was endolymphatic hydrops and excellent preservation of the organ of Corti and spiral ganglion cells. H & E stain. Mag. = 25×.

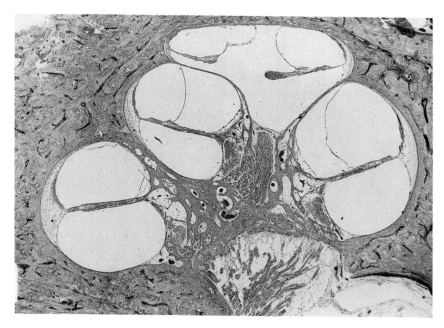

B

facial paralysis, vertigo, and sensorineural hearing loss. Auditory findings in patients suffering from hearing loss in this disorder suggested, at least in part, a primary neural lesion (Harbert & Young, 1967; Welsh & Welsh, 1962). Temporal bone histopathology of patients suffering hearing loss due to Ramsay Hunt syndrome demonstrated perivascular, perineural, and intraneural round cell aggregations in the auditory nerve and the modiolus (Blackley, Friedmann, & Wright, 1967). Although some cases demonstrated degeneration of the organ of Corti as well as of the auditory nerve, the histopathologic correlate of sensorineural loss was exclusively a neural degeneration in other cases. In addition, molecular pathologic studies (Wackym, 1997) have demonstrated by polymerase chain reaction (PCR) technology the varicella-zoster viral genome within the geniculate ganglion and perhaps the spiral ganglion cells, confirming the neurotropic characteristic of this virus and implicating primary neural disease as causative of the hearing loss. Occasionally, Ramsay Hunt syndrome may also involve other cranial nerves, including V, VI, IX, and X (Asnis, Micic, & Giaccio, 1996).

Cytomegalic Inclusion Disease

Cytomegalovirus (CMV) is part of the herpes virus group, *herpetoviridae*; it is a double-stranded DNA virus and may produce sensorineural

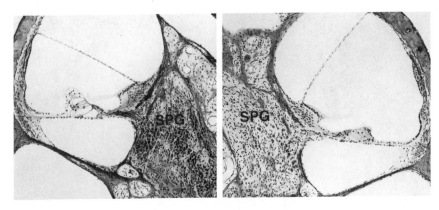

A

Figure 7–13. Experimental endolymphatic hydrops in the guinea pig. **A.** Midmodi-olar section of the apical turn of the cochlea demonstrated marked loss of spiral ganglion cells (SPG) on the hydropic side (right) compared with the normal spiral ganglion cell population on the control side (left). The hair cells of the organ of Corti were present bilaterally. H & E stain. Mag = 100×. **B.** Transmission electron micros-copy demonstrated evidence of degenerative change in the form of myelin figures among remaining spiral ganglion cells. Mag. = 6,100×. **C.** Among remaining den-dritic fibers there was evidence of degeneration including disorganization of the my-elin sheath, particularly at nodes of Ranvier (NR). Mag. = 11,000×.

hearing loss in children with congenital infection (Davis, 1979; Stagno, Pass, Dworsky, & Alford, 1983; Woolf, 1990). In congenital CMV infec-tion, permanent sequelae include multiple neurologic manifestations such as encephalitis, microencephaly, growth retardation, chorioretinitis, and hearing loss. Temporal bone findings suggested that in the inner ear, the cytomegalovirus may produce a generalized labyrinthitis, including coch-lear neurons (Strauss, 1990). Similar findings have been described in ex-perimental pathology in animal models (Harris, Fan, & Keithley, 1990).

CONCLUSIONS

In almost every etiology of sensorineural hearing loss in the human, there is degeneration of the auditory nerve, the central auditory pathways, or both. In most cases, the neural degeneration is secondary to pathology in the organ of Corti. Nonetheless, there is a significant number of causes of sensorineural hearing loss in which the principal histopathologic correlate is primary cochlear neuronal degeneration, which may be considered the equivalent of what has been called, in this text, auditory neuropathy.

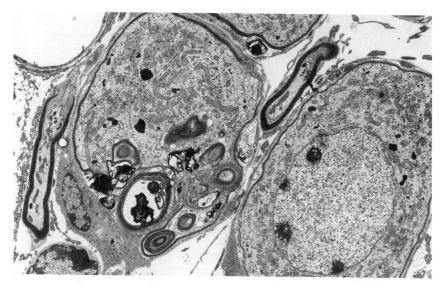

B

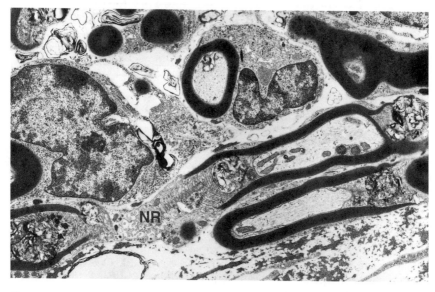

C

The range of processes that may produce primary cochlear neuronal degeneration include genetic, toxic, metabolic, immune-mediated, degenerative, and idiopathic diseases, and, finally, both fungal and viral infections. Primary cochlear neuronal degeneration—and by extension

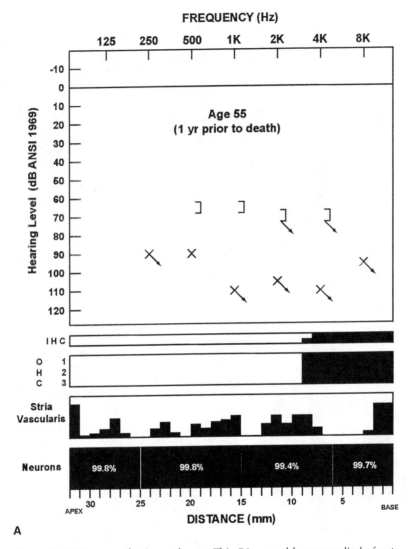

Figure 7–14. Paraneoplastic syndrome. This 56-year-old woman died of oat cell carcinoma of the lung. Three years before death, she developed dysphagia and progressive paralysis of muscles of the arms and neck. One year before death, she experienced sudden profound hearing loss in her left ear with disequilibrium. She had a mild sensorineural loss on the right. **A.** Cytocochleogram of the left ear. The principal histopathologic correlate of the profound sensorineural hearing loss was loss of spiral ganglion cells throughout the cochlea. **B.** Midmodiolar section of the left temporal bone. There was severe loss of spiral ganglion cells throughout the cochlea. H & E stain. Mag. = 25×. **C.** Photomicrograph of the basal turn of the cochlea. Although the organ of Corti was present, Rosenthal's canal (R) was almost totally devoid of spiral ganglion cells. H & E stain. Mag. = 60×.

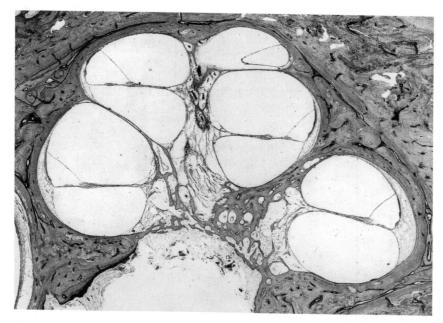

B

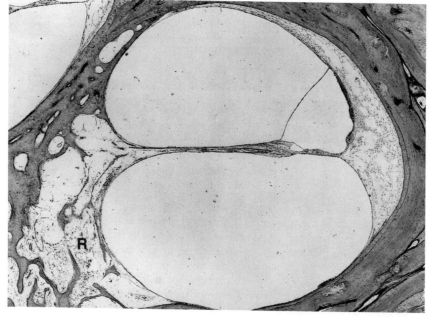

C

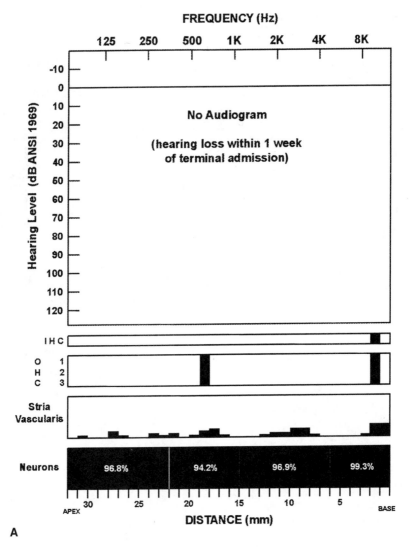

A

Figure 7–15. Fungal meningitis. This 60-year-old man died of cryptococcal meningitis. There was a 1-week history of hearing loss in the right ear; however, an audiogram was not performed before his death, 48 hours after hospital admission. **A.** Cytocochleogram of the right ear. Although the organ of Corti was largely intact, there was severe loss of spiral ganglion cells. **B.** Spiral ganglion in the basal turn of the right temporal bone. The outlines, or "ghosts," of degenerated cochlear neurons were seen throughout the spiral ganglion (arrows). There were many profiles of cryptococci (CC) within the spiral ganglion and within the internal auditory canal. H & E stain. Mag = 106×.

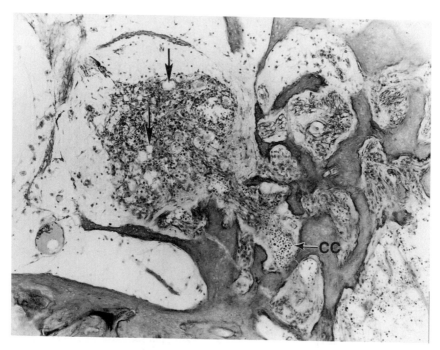

B

auditory neuropathy—is therefore not a disease, but a syndrome or phenotype that may be caused by a variety or a combination of disorders.

REFERENCES

Amantini, A., Rossi, L., DeSciosciolo, G., Bindi, A., Pagnini, P., & Zappoli, R. (1984). Auditory evoked potentials (early, middle, late components) and audiological tests in Friedreich's ataxia. *Electroencephalography and Clinical Neurophysiology, 58,* 37–47.

Anteunis, L. J., & Mooy, J. M. (1987). Hearing loss in a uraemic patient: Indications of involvement of the VIIIth nerve. *Journal of Laryngology and Otology, 101,* 492–496.

Asnis, D. S., Micic, L., & Giaccio, D. (1996). Ramsay Hunt syndrome presenting as a cranial polyneuropathy. *Cutis, 57,* 421–424.

Begeer, J. H., Scholte, F. A., & vanEssen, A. J. (1991). Two sisters with mental retardation, cataract, ataxia, progressive hearing loss, and polyneuropathy. *Journal of Medical Genetics, 28,* 884–885.

Belal, A., Jr. (1975). Usher's syndrome (Retinitis pigmentosa and deafness). A temporal bone report. *Journal of Laryngology and Otology, 89,* 175–181.

Bergamaschi, R., Romani, R., Zapoli, F., Versino, M., & Cosi, C. (1997). MRI and brain stem auditory evoked potential evidence of eighth cranial nerve involvement in multiple sclerosis. *Neurology, 48*, 270–272.

Blackley, B., Friedmann, I., & Wright, I. (1967). Herpes zoster auris associated with facial nerve palsy and auditory nerve symptoms. *Acta Otolaryngologica (Stockholm), 63*, 533–550.

Chance, P. F., & Fischbeck, K. H. (1994). Molecular genetics of Charcot-Marie-Tooth disease and related neuropathies. *Human Molecular Genetics, 3*, 1503–1507.

Chisin, R., Perlman, M., & Sohmer, H. (1979). Cochlear and brain stem responses in hearing loss following neonatal hyperbilirubinemia. *Annals of Otology, Rhinology and Laryngology, 88*, 352–357.

Citron, L., Dix, M. R., Hallpike, C. S., & Hood, J. D. (1963). A recent clinico-pathological study of cochlear nerve degeneration resulting from tumor pressure and disseminated sclerosis, with particular reference to the finding of normal threshold sensitivity for pure tones. *Acta Otolaryngologica (Stockholm), 56*, 330–337.

Davis, G. L. (1979). Congenital cytomegalovirus in hearing loss. Clinical and experimental observations. *Laryngoscope, 89*, 1681–1688.

Donovan, T. J. (1995). Mitochondrial encephalomyopathy: A rare genetic cause of sensorineural hearing loss. *Annals of Otology, Rhinology and Laryngology, 104*, 786–792.

Ell, J., Prasher, D., & Rudge, P. (1984). Neuro-otological abnormalities in Friedreich's ataxia. *Journal of Neurology, Neurosurgery and Psychiatry, 47*, 26–32.

Elverland, H. H., & Torbergsen, T. (1991). Audiologic findings in a family with mitochondrial disorder. *American Journal of Otolaryngology, 12*, 459–465.

Enander, A., & Stahle, J. (1967). Hearing in Meniere's disease. A study of pure-tone audiograms in 334 patients. *Acta Otolaryngologica (Stockholm), 64*, 543–546.

Ferrer, J. P., Biurrun, O., Lorente, J., Conget, J. I., deEspana, R., Esmatjes, E., & Gomis, R. (1991). Auditory function in young patients with type 1 diabetes mellitus. *Diabetes Research and Clinical Practice, 11*, 17–22.

Friedman, S. A., Schulman, R. H., & Weiss, S. (1975). Hearing and diabetic neuropathy. *Archives of Internal Medicine, 135*, 573–576.

Goodhill, V. (1967). Auditory pathway lesions resulting from Rh incompatibility. In F. McConnell & R. Ward (Eds.), *Deafness in childhood* (pp. 215–228). Nashville, TN: Vanderbilt University Press.

Hagemoser, K., Weinstein, J., Bresnick, G., Nellis, R., Kirkpatrick, S., & Pauli, R. M. (1989). Optic atrophy, hearing loss, and peripheral neuropathy. *American Journal of Medical Genetics, 33*, 61–65.

Hanft, K. L., & Haddad, J., Jr. (1994). Progressive sensorineural hearing loss (SNHL) and peripheral neuropathy: A case report. *International Journal of Pediatric Otorhinolaryngology, 28*, 229–234.

Harbert, F., & Young, I. M. (1967). Audiologic findings in Ramsay Hunt syndrome. *Archives of Otolaryngology, 85*, 632–639.

Harner, S. G. (1981). Hearing in adult onset diabetes mellitus. *Otolaryngology—Head & Neck Surgery, 89*, 322–327.

Harris, J. P., Fan, J. T., & Keithley, E. M. (1990). Immunologic responses in experimental cytomegalovirus labyrinthitis. *American Journal of Otolaryngology, 11*, 304–308.

Harrison, R. V. (1998, June). Cochlear frequency selectivity in animals with endo-lymphatic hydrops and in patients with Meniere's disease. In J. B. Nadol, Jr. (Ed.), *Second International Symposium on Meniere's Disease* (pp. 225–232). Amsterdam: Kugler and Ghedini Publications.

Harrison, R. V., & Prijs, V. F. (1984). Single cochlear fibre responses in guinea pigs with long term endolymphatic hydops. *Hearing Research, 14,* 79–84.

Hausler, R., & Levine, R. A. (1980). Brain stem auditory evoked potentials are related to interaural time discrimination in patients with multiple sclerosis. *Brain Research, 191,* 589–594.

Holmgren, L. (1964). Hearing tests in Meniere's disease. *Acta Otolaryngologica (Stockholm), Supplement, 192,* 115–120.

Igarashi, M., Weber, S. C., Alford, B. R., Coats, A. C., & Jerger, J. (1975). Temporal bone findings in cryptococcal meningitis. *Archives of Otolaryngology, 101,* 577–583.

Ishii, T., & Toriyama, M. (1977). Sudden deafness with severe loss of cochlear neurons. *Annals of Otology, Rhinology and Laryngology, 86,* 541–547.

Jin, H., May, M., Tranebjaerg, L., Kendall, E., Fontan, G., Jackson, J., Subramony, S. H., Arena, F., Lubs, H., Smith, S., Stevenson, R., Schwartz, C., & Vetrie, D. (1996). A novel X-linked gene, DDP, shows mutations in families with deafnesss (DFN–1), dystonia, mental deficiency and blindness. *Nature Genetics, 14,* 177–180.

Koehler, C. M., Leuenberger, D., Merchant, S., Renold, A., Junne, T., & Schatz, G. (1999). Human deafness dystonia syndrome is a mitochondrial disease. *Proceedings of the National Academy of Sciences of the United States of America, 96,* 2141–2146.

Lindsay, J. R., & Hinojosa, R. (1976). Histopathologic features of the inner ear associated with Kearns-Sayre syndrome. *Archives of Otolaryngology, 102,* 747–752.

Lindsay, J. R., Kohut, R. I., & Sciarra, P. A. (1967). Meniere's disease: Pathology and manifestations. *Annals of Otology, Rhinology and Laryngology, 76,* 5–22.

Lounsbury-Martin, B. L., Martin, G. K., Coats, A. C., & Johnson, K. C. (1988, June). Alternations in acoustic-distortion products and cochlear nerve-fiber activity in hydropic rabbits. In J. B. Nadol, Jr. (Ed.), *Second International Symposium on Meniere's Disease* (pp. 337–350). Amsterdam: Kugler and Ghedini Publications.

Maurer, K., Schafer, E., Hopf, H. C., & Leitner, H. (1980). The location by early auditory evoked potentials (EAEP) of acoustic nerve and brain stem demyelinization in multiple sclerosis (MS). *Journal of Neurology, 223,* 43–58.

McGill, T. J. (1978). Mycotic infection of the temporal bone. *Archives of Otolaryngology, 104,* 140–144.

Meurman, O. H., & Grahne, B. (1956). Hearing and Meniere's disease. *Practica Oto-Rhino-Laryngologica, 18,* 365–376.

Musiek, F. E., Weider, D. J., & Mueller, R. J. (1982). Audiologic findings in Charcot-Marie-Tooth disease. *Archives of Otolaryngology, 108,* 595-599.

Nadol, J. B., Jr. (1978). Hearing loss as a sequela of meningitis. *Laryngoscope, 88,* 739–755.

Nadol, J. B., Jr. (1979). Electron microscopic findings in presbycusic degeneration of the basal turn of the human cochlea. *Otolaryngology—Head & Neck Surgery, 87,* 818–836.

Nadol, J. B., Jr. (1988a). Innervation densities of inner and outer hair cells of the human organ of Corti. Evidence for auditory neural degeneration in a case of Usher's syndrome. *ORL Journal of Oto-Rhinolaryngol and Its Related Specialties, 50,* 363–370.

Nadol, J. B., Jr. (1988b). Application of electron microscopy to human otopathology. Ultrastructural findings in neural presbycusis, Meniere's disease and Usher's syndrome. *Acta Otolaryngologica (Stockholm), 105,* 411–419.

Nadol, J. B., Jr., Adams, J. C., & Kim, J. R. (1995). Degenerative changes in the organ of Corti and lateral cochlear wall in experimental endolymphatic hydrops in human Meniere's disease. *Acta Otolaryngologica (Stockholm), Supplement 519,* 47–59.

Nadol, J. B., Jr., & Thornton, A. R. (1987). Ultrastrctural findings in a case of Meniere's disease. *Annals of Otology, Rhinology and Laryngology, 96,* 449–454.

Nwaesei, C. G., VanAerde, J., Boyden, M., & Perlman, M. (1984). Changes in auditory brainstem responses in hyperbilirubinemic infants before and after exchange transfusion. *Pediatrics, 74,* 800–803.

Oshima, T., Ueda, N., Ikeda, K., Abe, K., & Takasaka, T. (1996). Bilateral sensorineural hearing loss associated with the point mutation in mitochondrial genome. *Laryngoscope, 106,* 43–48.

Ouvrier, R. (1996). Correlation between the histopathologic, genotypic, and phenotypic features of hereditary peripheral neuropathies in childhood. *Journal of Child Neurology, 11,* 133–146.

Pareyson, D., Scaioli, V., Berta, E., & Sghirlanzoni, A. (1995). Acoustic nerve in peripheral neuropathy: A BAEP study. Brainstem auditory evoked potentials. *Electromyography and Clinical Neurophysiology, 35,* 359–364.

Perlman, M., Fainmesser, P., Sohmer, H., Tamari, H., Wax, Y., & Pevsmer, B. (1983). Auditory nerve-brainstem evoked responses in hyperbilirubinemic neonates. *Pediatrics, 72,* 658–664.

Quine, D. B., Regan, D., & Murray, T. J. (1984). Degraded discrimination between speech-like sounds by patients with multiple sclerosis and Friedreich's ataxia. *Brain, 107,* 1113–1122.

Raglan, E., Prasher, D. K., Trinder, E., & Rudge, P. (1987). Auditory function in hereditary motor and sensory neuropathy (Charcot-Marie-Tooth disease). *Acta Otolaryngologica (Stockholm), 103,* 50–55.

Rybak, L. P. (1992). Hearing: The effects of chemicals. *Otolaryngology—Head & Neck Surgery, 106,* 677–686.

Satya-Murti, S., Cacace, A. T., & Hanson, P. A. (1979). Abnormal auditory evoked potentials in hereditary motor-sensory neuropathy. *Annals of Neurology, 5,* 445–448.

Satya-Murti, S., Cacace, A., & Hanson, P. (1980). Auditory dysfunction in Friedreich ataxia: Result of spiral ganglion degeneration. *Neurology, 30,* 1047–1053.

Schuknecht, H. F. (1964). Further observations of the pathology of presbycusis. *Archives of Otolaryngology, 80,* 369–382.

Schuknecht, H. F. (1975). Pathophysiology of Meniere's disease. *Otolaryngologic Clinics of North America, 8,* 507–514.

Schuknecht, H. F. (1993). *Pathology of the ear* (2nd ed.). Philadelphia: Lea and Febiger.

Schuknecht, H. F., Benitez, J. T., & Beekhuis, J. (1962). Further observations on the pathology of Meniere's disease. *Annals of Otology, Rhinology and Laryngology, 71,* 1039–1053.

Schuknecht, H. F., & Donovan, E. D. (1986). The pathology of idiopathic sudden sensorineural hearing loss. *Archives of Otorhinolaryngology, 243,* 1–15.

Schuknecht, J. F., & Nadol, J. B., Jr. (1994). Temporal bone pathology in a case of Cogan's syndrome. *Laryngoscope, 104,* 1335–1342.

Shanon, E., Himelfarb, M. Z., & Gold, S. (1981). Auditory function of Friedreich's ataxia. Electrophysiologic study of a family. *Archives of Otolaryngology, 107,* 254–256.

Shapiro, S. M., & Hecox, K. E. (1989). Brain stem auditory evoked potentials in jaundiced Gunn rats. *Annals of Otology, Rhinology and Laryngology, 98,* 308–317.

Shinkawa, H., & Nadol, J. B., Jr. (1986). Histopathology of the inner ear in Usher's syndrome as observed by light and electron microscopy. *Annals of Otology, Rhinology and Laryngology, 95,* 313–318.

Smith, T. W., Bhawan, J., Keller, R. B., & DeGirolami, U. (1980). Charcot-Marie-Tooth disease associated with hypertrophic neuropathy: A neuropathologic study of two cases. *Journal of Neuropathology and Experimental Neurology, 39,* 420–440.

Spitzer, J. B. (1981). Auditory effects of chronic alcoholism. *Drug and Alcohol Dependence, 4,* 317–335.

Spoendlin, H. (1974). Optic cochleovestibular degenerations in hereditary ataxias. II. Temporal bone pathology in two cases of Friedreich's ataxia with vestibulocochlear disorders. *Brain, 97,* 41–48.

Stagno, S., Pass, R. F., Dworsky, M. E., & Alford, C. A. (1983). Congenital and perinatal cytomegalovirus infections. *Seminars in Perinatology, 7,* 31–42.

Stahle, J. (1976). Advanced Meniere's disease. A study of 356 severely disabled patients. *Acta Otolaryngologica (Stockholm), 81,* 113–119.

Starr, A., Picton, T. W., Sininger, Y. S., Hood, L. J., & Berlin, C. I. (1996). Auditory neuropathy. *Brain, 119,* 741–753.

Strauss, M. (1990). Human cytomegalovirus labyrinthitis. *American Journal of Otolaryngology, 11,* 292–298.

Taylor, M. J., McMenamin, J. B., Andermann, E., & Waters, G. V. (1982). Electrophysiological investigation of the auditory system in Friedreich's ataxia. *Canadian Journal of Neurological Science, 9,* 131–135.

Uchino, M., Okajima, T., Eto, K., Kumamoto, T., Mishima, I., & Ando, M. (1995). Neurologic features of chronic Minamata disease (organic mercury poisoning) certified at autopsy. *Internal Medicine, 34,* 744–747.

Uziel, A., Marot, M., & Pujol, R. (1983). The Gunn rat: An experimental model for central deafness. *Acta Otolaryngologica (Stockholm), 95,* 651–656.

Wackym, P. A. (1997). Molecular temporal bone pathology II: Ramsay Hunt syndrome, Herpes Zoster Oticus. *Laryngoscope, 107,* 1165–1175.

Welsh, L. W., & Welsh, J. J. (1962). Herpes zoster involving the head and neck. *Laryngoscope, 72,* 653–663.

Woolf, N. K. (1990). Experimental congenital cytomegalovirus labyrinthitis and sensorineural hearing loss. *American Journal of Otolaryngology, 11,* 299–301.

Wright, A., & Dyck, P. J. (1995). Hereditary sensory neuropathy with sensorineural deafness and early-onset dementia. *Neurology, 45* Pt 1, 560–562.

Wu, M. F., Ison, J. R., Wecker, J. R., & Lapham, L. W. (1985). Cutaneous and auditory function in rats following methyl mercury poisoning. *Toxicology and Applied Pharmacology, 79,* 377–388.

Yamasoba, T., Oka, Y., Tsukuda, K., Nakamura, M., & Kaga, K. (1996). Auditory findings in patients with maternally inherited diabetes and deafness harboring a point mutation in the mitochondrial transfer RNA$^{Leu(UUR)}$ gene. *Laryngoscope, 106,* 49–54.

Yoshikawa, H., Nishimura, T., Nakatsuji, Y., Fujimura, H., Himoro, M., Hayasaka, K., Sakoda, S., & Yanagihara, T. (1994). Elevated expression of messenger RNA for peripheral myelin protein 22 in biopsied peripheral nerves of patients with Charcot-Marie-Tooth disease type 1A. *Annals of Neurology, 35,* 445–450.

Zimmermann, C. E., Burgess, B. J., & Nadol, J. B. (1995). Patterns of degeneration in the human cochlear nerve. *Hearing Research, 90,* 192–201.

8

Psychoacoustics and Speech Perception in Auditory Neuropathy

Fan-Gang Zeng, Sandy Oba, Smita Garde,
Yvonne Sininger, and Arnold Starr

Auditory neuropathy (AN) is typically associated with hearing loss, the presence of otoacoustic emissions, and the absence of evoked potentials. Functional deficits in people with this disorder are poorly appreciated, however. They often demonstrate a speech recognition deficit, particularly in noise, that is disproportional to the amount of pure-tone hearing loss if it were sensory in nature. Conventional hearing aids are less effective than expected in alleviating their speech recognition problems in daily life. The causes of AN are not clear and may be related to mechanical, chemical, or neuronal deficiency (or a combination of these factors) in the inner hair cell, the synapse between the inner hair cell and the auditory neurons, or the auditory neurons (Harrison, 1998; Starr, Picton, Sininger, Hood, & Berlin, 1996). This chapter describes a psychophysical approach to the description of functional processing deficits in AN.

There are three goals in psychophysical studies of AN. The first is to characterize the functional capabilities in people with auditory neuropathy. The emphasis here is to understand why these people often complain that they can hear sounds but cannot understand speech. The second goal is to develop behavioral tests that can help delineate underlying physiological mechanisms and differentiate hearing loss of different origins (e.g., damage to outer hair cells, inner hair cells, and the auditory nerve). The third goal in psychophysical studies of auditory neuropathy is to provide guidance for designing auditory prostheses and rehabilitation strategies that best fit the residual processing capabilities in these people.

We have collected extensive psychophysical data for intensity, frequency, and temporal processing in subjects diagnosed with AN. Our results indicate that although there are abnormalities in intensity and frequency processing, the impaired temporal processing is likely the major reason for the poor speech recognition in AN subjects. This conclusion receives further support from a simulation of the temporal processing impairment in listeners with normal hearing who can produce psychophysical and speech recognition deficits similar to those seen in AN subjects.

SPECIFIC STUDIES

Subjects

We studied 10 AN subjects, including one with unilateral neuropathy. We also studied three control subjects including (a) the healthy ear in the subject with unilateral neuropathy, (b) one subject with cochlear impairment who has an atypical low-frequency hearing loss configuration, and (c) a group of six subjects with normal hearing, including three female and three male subjects, ages 27 to 35 years old; all had pure-tone air- and bone-conduction thresholds of 20 dB HL or better for the octave frequencies between 250 and 8000 Hz.

Table 8–1 lists audiologic and neurologic test results of the subjects with AN and of control subjects. Figure 8–1 shows pure-tone thresholds as a function of frequency for the subjects with AN and the control subjects. The subjects with AN exhibited a wide range of hearing loss; on average, they had a moderate (60 dB) hearing loss in the low frequencies but only a mild hearing loss (30–40 dB) in the high frequencies. Subjects with AN had normal measures of cochlear outer hair cell functions (i.e., otoacoustic emissions, cochlear microphonics, or both were present in all subjects). No subjects with AN demonstrated wave I on auditory brain stem potentials, and all who were tested showed absent acoustic middle ear muscle reflexes to tones up to and including 110 dB HL. Brain imaging results were normal in the six subjects with AN who were tested. The control ear from the subject with a unilateral auditory neuropathy (N-AN8) had normal pure-tone thresholds, present otoacoustic emissions, cochlear microphonics, auditory brain stem potentials, and 100%-correct word recognition.

The subject with cochlear impairment in this study had a low-frequency hearing loss and near-normal hearing at higher frequencies. This configuration was chosen to mimic the loss of average auditory neuropathy subjects and was different from the usual high-frequency-sloping hearing loss typically seen in subjects with cochlear loss. His

Table 8–1. Audiologic and neurologic test results of subjects with auditory neuropathy and control subjects.

Subject	Age	Gender	PTA (dB)	Speech (%)	Otoacoustic Emission (dB)	Cochlear Microphonic	ABR	Acoustic Reflex	Imaging	PN
AN1	50	F	32	56	TEOAE = 11.8	Present	Abnormal	Absent	DNT	Yes
AN2	53	F	15	DNT	TEOAE = 8.9	DNT	Abnormal	DNT	DNT	Yes
AN3	19	F	72	12	DPOAE = 3–15	DNT	Absent	Absent	Normal MRI	Yes
AN4	23	F	38	0	TEOAE = 5.4	Present	Absent	Absent	Normal MRI	No
AN5	17	F	62	0	Absent	Present	Absent	Absent	Normal CT	No
AN6	37	M	55	CNT	DPOAE = 4–13	DNT	Absent	Absent	Normal MRI	Yes
AN7	27	M	45	40	TEOAE = 12.3	Present	Abnormal	Absent	DNT	No
AN8	10	M	82	0	DPOAE = 3–10	Present	Abnormal	DNT	DNT	No
AN9	13	M	63	0	TEOAE = 12.6	Present	Absent	Absent	Normal	No
AN10	22	M	30	64	TEOAE = 11.7	DNT	Absent	DNT	Normal PET	No
Average	27.1		49.4	21.5						
CHL	40	F	60	84	DPOAE = 5 dB @ 6,000 only	DNT	Present	DNT	DNT	No
N-AN8	10	M	7	100	TEOAE = 10.3	Present	Present	DNT	DNT	No

Note. F = female; M = male; PTA = pure-tone average threshold at 500, 1000, and 2000 Hz; CNT = could not test; DNT = did not test; TEOAE = transient-evoked otoacoustic emission; DPOAE = distortion product otoacoustic emission; ABR = auditory brain stem response; MRI = magnetic resonance imaging; CT = computer tomography; PET = positron emission tomography; PN = peripheral neuropathy.

AUDIOGRAM

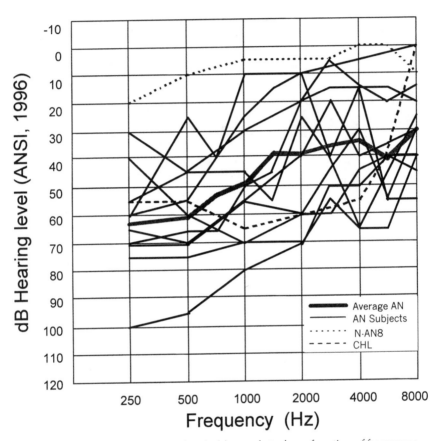

Figure 8–1. Audiogram. Pure-tone thresholds are plotted as a function of frequency. Narrow lines indicate individual subjects with auditory neuropathy, and the wide line indicates the average of these subjects. The long dashed line indicates the control subject with a cochlear hearing loss, and the dotted line indicates normal ear of the unilateral auditory neuropathy case (N–AN8).

low-frequency hearing loss generally was within 20 dB of the average hearing thresholds of AN subjects. The subject with cochlear impairment had no otoacoustic emissions except at the 6000 Hz where the hearing threshold was normal, and all components of the auditory brain stem potential were identified. His 84% word recognition was consistent with his moderate pure-tone loss. In contrast, word recognition scores among subjects with AN ranged from 0 to 64% with an average of 22%—

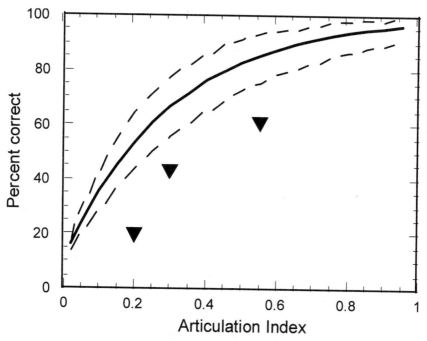

Figure 8–2. Articulation index (AI) analysis on speech recognition deficits in people with auditory neuropathy. The solid line and surrounding dashed lines indicate the expected relationship between AI (abscissa) and speech discrimination scores (ordinate) as determined by Dubno and Alstrom (1995). The actual relationships for three subjects with auditory neuropathy are indicated by the closed triangle symbols.

significantly lower than what would be expected from their pure-tone hearing loss. Figure 8–2 shows an estimate of the phoneme recognition scores that should be expected from the pure-tone threshold measurement (Dubno & Ahlstrom, 1995). A simplified version of the articulation index (AI; Mueller & Killion, 1990) was applied to the phoneme recognition scores of three subjects with auditory neuropathy. This showed that the actual phoneme recognition scores of these subjects were at least two standard deviations poorer than the AI-predicted scores.

Stimuli

In the intensity and frequency processing experiments, tonal stimuli of 200 ms in duration were generated digitally using TDT System II (Tucker-Davis Technology). In the temporal processing experiments, a broadband

(20–14,000 Hz) white noise was generated and controlled digitally to measure temporal integration, gap detection, and temporal modulation transfer functions. The noise had a duration of 500 ms and 2.5-ms cosine-squared ramps. In the gap detection experiment, a silent interval was produced in the center of the noise. In the temporal modulation function experiment, the same 500-ms noise was presented at a maximum comfortable level determined for each subject (ranging from 29 to 77 dB SL). For the modulated signals, the presentation level was dynamically adjusted to achieve the same root-mean-square level (given the amount of modulation) as the unmodulated stimuli.

Figure 8–3 shows the flow chart for the stimuli generated for simulating auditory neuropathy in the listeners with normal hearing. The neuropathy simulation algorithm divided a speech signal into 16 third-octave bands and extracted the band-specific temporal envelope by half-wave rectification and low-pass filtering (Drullman, Festen, & Plomp, 1994). The low-pass filters were designed according to the measured temporal modulation transfer functions and covered four degrees of temporal processing impairment found in the present neuropathy subjects: mild (modulation peak sensitivity = –17 dB and 3 dB cutoff = 100 Hz), moderate (–14 dB and 50 Hz), severe (–8 dB and 25 Hz), and profound (–2 dB and 15 Hz). The low-pass-filtered temporal envelopes were used to modulate the amplitude of the fine-structure of the original acoustic signal, resulting in a temporally smeared acoustic waveform.

Procedure

We used standard procedures to collect and analyze all audiologic and neurologic data. Pure-tone averaged thresholds were based on thresholds at frequencies of 500, 1000, and 2000 Hz. Word recognition was based on NU–6 (1/2 list) test materials. This word test could not be performed on subject AN6 because of his nonnative English-speaking status. Auditory brain stem responses were recorded between vertex and the stimulated ear and identified as either absent (no definable waveforms) or abnormal (presence of only wave V). Acoustic reflexes were measured for pure-tone stimuli at 500, 1000, 2000, and 4000 Hz, presented ipsilaterally, contralaterally, or both to the stimulated ear using a Grason-Stadler GSI 33 middle ear analyzer. Otoacoustic emissions were measured with a V5 ILO92 OAE system by Otodynamics Ltd. and reported as the dB value above the noise floor. The cochlear microphonic was measured from auditory brain stem responses averaged to separate presentations of condensation and rarefaction clicks. All psychophysical tests used a three-alternative, forced-choice procedure to measure the threshold that resulted in a 70.7% correct response.

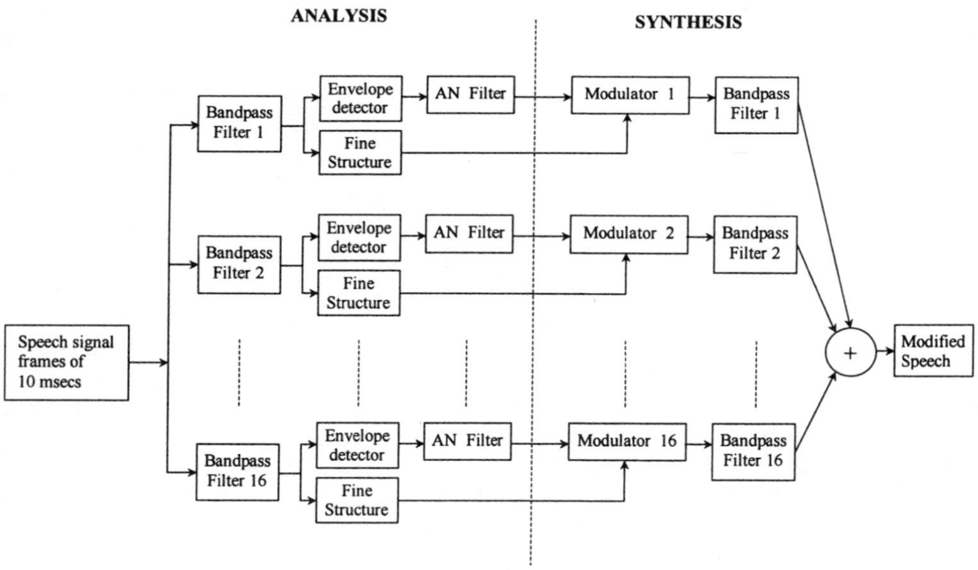

Figure 8–3. Signal processing chart for simulations of auditory neuropathy. The degree of auditory neuropathy was based on temporal modulation transfer functions (see text and the table on the left). Because normal-hearing listeners had a peak sensitivity of −20 dB and mild neuropathy subjects had a peak sensitivity of −17 dB, a 3-dB attenuation was applied to the temporal envelope signals in the simulation. Examples of simulations can be found on the following Web site: http://www.com.uci.edu/hesp/simulations.html#neuropathy.

AN Filters:

Degree of Auditory Neuropathy	Cutoff frequency (Hz)	Gain (db)
Normal	238 Hz	0db
Mild	100 Hz	-3 db
Moderate	50 Hz	-6 db
Severe	25 Hz	-12 db
Profound	15 Hz	-18 db

RESULTS

Experiments were conducted to identify the nature of loudness growth, intensity discrimination, frequency discrimination, temporal integration, gap detection, and temporal modulation transfer function in subjects with AN. An acoustic simulation of speech perception was developed based on the measured psychophysical data in auditory neuropathy subjects. The simulation produced similarly impaired temporal and speech processing results in subjects with normal hearing. Data in temporal processing from eight subjects were reported previously (Zeng, Oba, Garde, Sininger, & Starr, 1999).

Psychophysical Measures in Auditory Neuropathy

Intensity Processing

We collected loudness growth measures in one subject (AN10) and intensity discrimination in four subjects with AN. Figure 8–4 shows loudness growth measured by two different methods. The left panel shows loudness growth functions at 250, 1000, and 4000 Hz measured by absolute magnitude estimation. The dashed lines indicate the best fit to the data using a power function (Zwislocki, 1965), where n is the exponent of the power function and r is the regression coefficient. The threshold (indicated by arrows) for the 250, 1000, and 4000-Hz tone was 71, 17, and 17 dB SPL, respectively. Loudness growth at 1000 Hz in listeners with normal hearing is depicted as the solid line (Hellman and Zwislocki, 1963). Although it appears that the subject shifted his internal scale for the 4000-Hz tone (an overall vertical shift in the numbers), he demonstrated a much more compressive loudness function ($n = 0.06$ to 0.10) than did the normal control subjects ($n = 0.27$) at all three test frequencies.

The right panel in Figure 8–4 shows loudness scaling data using the identical approach to that by Allen et al. (1990). Because loudness scaling is not a ratio scale, only qualitative information on loudness growth can be inferred. Still, the general compressive trend can be viewed in the scaling data (for the 1000- and 4000-Hz tones with normal threshold): low-level tones in this subject were judged louder than that by the normal controls, whereas high-level tones were judged softer. At 250 Hz, loudness recruitment was observed.

Figure 8–5 shows intensity discrimination data collected in four subjects with AN and the normal control subjects (the area between dashed lines represents the mean plus and minus two standard deviations). These data show that although intensity discrimination was worse at low sensation levels in two of the four subjects with AN it was generally in the normal range. Because subjects with AN often have problems in speech

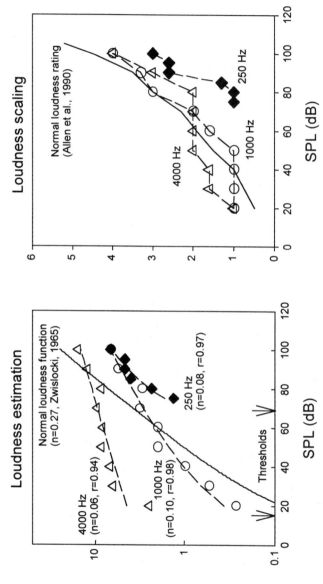

Figure 8–4. Loudness growth in one subject with neuropathy (AN10). Normal loudness growth is indicated by the solid line.

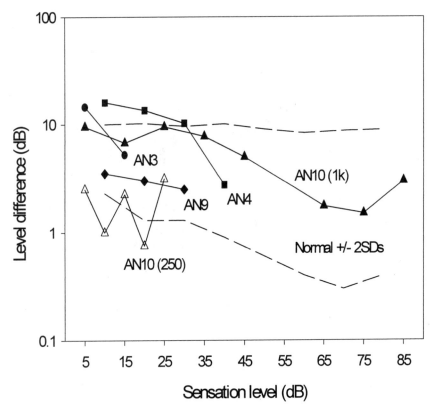

Figure 8–5. Intensity discrimination in subjects with normal hearing (mean ± 2 SD, marked by dashed lines) and in four subjects with neuropathy (symbols and solid lines).

recognition even if the speech was presented at high levels, the present intensity discrimination data suggest that intensity processing is not a major factor contributing to their speech recognition problems.

Frequency Processing

Figure 8–6 shows frequency discrimination in three subjects with auditory neuropathy and normal control subjects (mean ±2 standard deviations). For listeners with normal hearing, the difference limen (y-axis) increases as a monotonic function of frequency (x-axis). They require several Hz to notice a difference in pitch for frequencies less than 1000 Hz and several hundreds of Hz at 8000 Hz. Interestingly, the three subjects with auditory neuropathy showed a totally different pattern of results; the difference

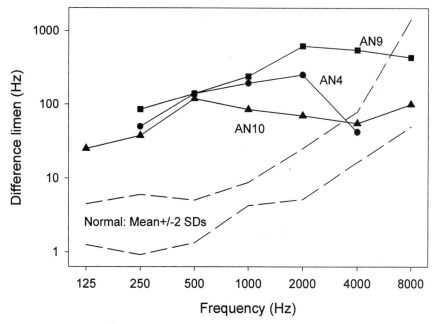

Figure 8–6. Frequency discrimination in subjects with normal hearing (mean ± 2 SD, marked by dashed lines) and in three subjects with neuropathy (symbols and solid lines).

limen was a nonmonotonic function of frequency. Their difference limens were much poorer than those of the control subjects with normal hearing at low frequencies (< 2000 Hz) but continued to improve as a function of frequency, finally becoming indistinguishable from the normal values at high frequencies (> 4000 Hz). The poor frequency discrimination in the middle frequency region (1000–3000 Hz) may pose some problem for discerning the second formant frequencies of two spectrally closely spaced vowels but should not prevent subjects with AN from distinguishing other speech sounds, such as fricatives, in which spectral cues are not as fine as the vowels. If we believe that the synchronous neural activity is disrupted in AN, the present data should provide an interesting demonstration on the role of temporal cues in pitch encoding for low frequencies (< 2000 Hz).

Temporal Processing

Figure 8–7 shows that detection thresholds for listeners with normal hearing (the shaded area) decrease at a rate of about 3 dB per doubling of

TEMPORAL INTEGRATION

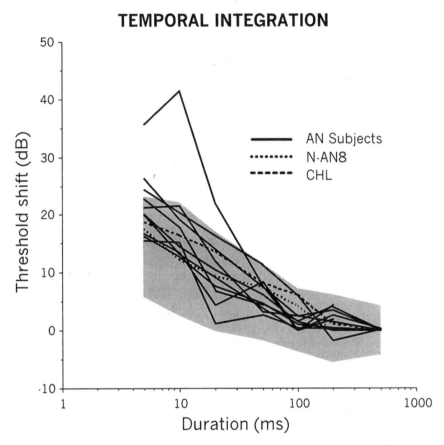

Figure 8–7. Temporal integration functions. Threshold shifts (y-axis) refer to the difference in dB between detection thresholds for noise bursts of different durations (x-axis) and that for the detection threshold at the longest duration (500 ms). Normal control data are represented as the shaded area (mean ± 2 SD). Neuropathy data are represented by solid lines. The dashed line represents the cochlear-impaired case, and the dotted line represents the healthy ear of the unilateral case.

signal duration for durations up to 100–200 milliseconds. Figure 8–7 also shows (with the exception of AN3, the original case in the Starr et al. 1991 study) that subjects with AN, as well as the two control subjects, showed normal or nearly normal temporal integration functions. Although subject AN3 had a much steeper slope of −8 dB, the remaining nine subjects with AN had an averaged slope of −4 dB, much closer to the normal value. Thus, the results from the detection of short-duration sounds apparently could not explain the poor speech recognition in subjects with neuropathy.

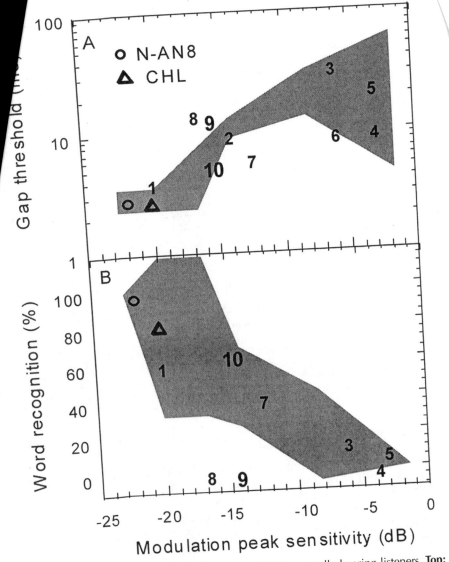

Figure 8–10. Simulations of auditory neuropathy in normally hearing listeners. **Top:** Gap detection thresholds at 40 dB SL. The gap detection threshold is plotted as a function of the severity of the auditory neuropathy, represented as the peak sensitivity of the temporal modulation transfer function (x-axis). The shaded area represents the mean ± 2 SD from normally hearing listeners who performed gap detection by listening to temporally smeared waveforms (see text for details). The digits denote gap detection thresholds measured for each of the subjects with auditory neuropathy also tested at 40 dB SL (from Figure 8–8). The symbols denote two control subjects (also from Figure 8–8). Because the listeners with normal hearing and the two control subjects all produced peak sensitivity values of about –20 dB, their x-coordinates were shifted by 1–2 dB to avoid overlap. **Bottom:** Word recognition from listeners with normal hearing who listened to both unprocessed words and temporally smeared speech sounds simulating various degrees of auditory neuropathy (see text for details). Symbols are identical to that in Figure 8–10A.

GAP DETECTION

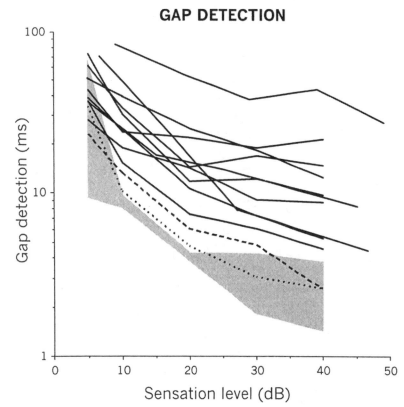

Figure 8–8. Gap detection thresholds. Detection thresholds (y-axis) are plotted as a function of sound presentation level (dB SL). Normal control data are represented as the shaded area (mean ± 2 SD). Neuropathy data are represented by solid lines. The dashed line represents the cochlear-impaired case, and the dotted line represents the healthy ear of the unilateral case.

Figure 8–8, on the other hand, shows that detecting short, silent intervals, or gaps, in acoustic signals was uniformly impaired in the subjects with AN. In both the listeners with normal hearing (shaded area) and the unilateral control, gap detection thresholds improved from 20–30 ms at low sound levels to 2–3 ms at high sound levels. The subject with cochlear impairment had slightly elevated gap detection thresholds at moderate sound levels but reached the normal range of values at the highest sound level, a pattern similar to previous studies employing listeners with cochlear impairment (Fitzgibbons & Gordon-Salant, 1987; Florentine & Buus, 1984; Moore & Glasberg, 1988). In contrast, all subjects with AN still had large deficits at the highest sound level; their gap detection thresholds were 2 to 25 times greater than normal.

TEMPORAL MODULATION TRANSFER FUNCTION

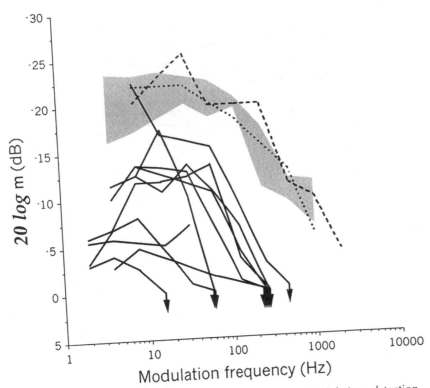

Figure 8–9. Temporal modulation transfer functions. Modulation detection thresholds (y-axis) represented as 20*log*(m) are plotted as a function of modulation frequency (x-axis). Arrows represent the fact that subjects could not reliably detect the presence of even a 100% modulated noise. Normal control data are represented as the shaded area (mean ± 2 SD). Neuropathy data are represented by solid lines. The dashed line represents the cochlear-impaired case, and the dotted line represents the healthy ear of the unilateral case.

Figure 8–9 shows the measured sensitivity to slow and fast temporal fluctuations (i.e., modulation transfer functions, see Viemeister, 1979). We modeled the modulation transfer function as a first-order Butterworth low-pass filter (Table 8–2). The listeners with normal hearing showed a low-pass function, being most sensitive (peak sensitivity = –20.4 dB) to slow temporal fluctuations and becoming less sensitive as the fluctuation rate was increased (3 dB cutoff frequency = 247 Hz). Both the unilateral and control subjects with cochlear impairment showed modulation transfer functions that were virtually indistinguishable from the normal

Table 8–2. Summary of temporal modulation transfer functio.

Subjects	Sensation Level (dB)	Peak Sensitivity (dB)	
Normal hearing	40	−20.4	2.
CHL	37	−21.8	23·
N-AN8	41	−21.6	175.
AN1	40	−20.1	41.7
AN2	29	−13.8	51.2
AN3	49	−5.8	32.9
AN4	40	−3.6	106.6
AN5	42	−3.6	14.1
AN6	45	−6.1	44.8
AN7	39	−12.4	72.3
AN8	40	−16.4	14.3
AN9	40	−12.9	38.8
AN10	77	−12.9	38.8
Average	44.1	−10.8	45.6

Note. Sensation level refers to the dB value of the noise presentation level above the subject's absolute hearing threshold for the same noise stimulus. Peak sensitivity and 3-dB cutoff frequency were estimated using a first-order Butterworth filter. The coefficient (*r*) reflects the goodness of fit. A different model (Formby & Muir, 1988) that has a −3 dB per octave slope was also evaluated and yielded generally higher peak sensitivity values (ranging from −3.9 to −23.1 dB) and lower cutoff frequencies (ranging from 4 Hz to 120 Hz). The goodness of fit of this model (*r* = .72–.98) was slightly worse than the first-order Butterworth filter.

low-pass function. In contrast, all subjects with AN showed impaired sensitivity to both slow and fast temporal fluctuations. The average peak sensitivity at low modulation frequencies was –10.8 dB and the average 3-dB cutoff modulation frequency was 45.6 Hz. These values were about one third (–10.8 vs. –20.4 dB) and one fifth (45.6 vs. 247 Hz), respectively, of the corresponding values obtained for our control listeners.

Simulations of AN

The temporal modulation transfer function measured for the subjects with AN allowed development of simulations of auditory neuropathy in listeners with normal hearing (Drullman et al., 1994). The detailed method of simulation was described earlier (see Figure 8–3). Figure 8–10 (top panel) shows simulation results of gap detection thresholds, which increased monotonically from about 2–20 ms as the severity of the simulated AN was increased from "mild" to "profound." The actual gap thresholds from subjects with AN generally were within two standard deviations of the

simulated thresholds. For comparison, the two control conditions also are shown for the healthy ear of the unilateral patient with AN (circle) and for the listener with cochlear impairment (triangle).

Figure 8–10 (bottom panel) shows results of simulated word recognition, which decreased monotonically to a 50%-correct level when the modulation detection threshold was elevated by about 5 dB from the normal value of –20 dB and reached 0%-correct level with about 15 dB elevations. Actual word recognition scores from eight neuropathy and two control subjects are shown in the same fashion as in the top panel of Figure 8–10. With two exceptions (AN8 and AN9), poor word recognition was consistent with the degree of impaired temporal processing in neuropathy subjects. The exceptional subjects had more severe hearing loss, suggesting that additional factors such as audibility may have contributed to the poor speech recognition in these two subjects. Adding audibility to modulation measures (temporal factors) allows excellent prediction of word recognition in patients with auditory neuropathy. The following equation reveals an $r = .93$ and $p = .01$.

$$word\% = 49.5 - .99 * PTA - 2.02 * TMTF(dB) + 0.04 * TMTF(Hz)$$

where PTA is pure-tone-averaged threshold and TMTF represents measures in temporal modulation transfer functions.

DISCUSSION

The present tests have revealed a severe temporal processing impairment in subjects with auditory neuropathy, in contrast to the relatively normal temporal processing often associated with hearing disorders due to cochlear damage (Bacon & Gleitman, 1992; Bacon & Viemeister, 1985; Fitzgibbons & Gordon-Salant, 1987; Florentine & Buus, 1984; Formby & Muir, 1988; Moore & Glasberg, 1988; Moore, Shailer, & Schooneveldt, 1992). To assess whether a lack of audibility is a confounding factor, a correlation was computed between subjects' averaged pure-tone thresholds (column 4 in Table 8–1) and their peak sensitivities to slow fluctuations (column 3 in Table 8–2). Only an insignificant correlation ($r = .23$) was found between the pure-tone average threshold and the peak sensitivity. In addition, a high-pass filter at 1000 Hz (135 dB/octave) was applied to simulate the low-frequency hearing loss in a subject with normal hearing. This produced no significant effect on modulation transfer functions (–17 vs. –16 dB, –19 vs. –19 dB, –17 vs. –17 dB, –17 vs. –18 dB at modulation frequencies 4, 8, 16, 32 Hz, respectively). These analyses suggest a true temporal processing deficit in AN, rather than a byproduct of hearing loss due to limited bandwidths at low sensation levels. This conclusion received additional support from the simulation results that the degree of temporal processing impairment can account for the abnormal speech recognition observed in subjects with neuropathy. The present finding of a close coupling between temporal and speech processing deficits complements the recent emphasis on speech recognition using temporal cues in general (e.g., Shannon, Zeng, Wygonski, Kamath, & Ekelid, 1995; Van Tasell, Soli, Kirby, & Widin, 1987) and amplitude modulations in particular (Arai & Greenberg, 1998; Greenberg & Arai, 1998).

Desynchronous Neural Activity

Although the exact physiologic process underlying AN is not clear, there is evidence linking the observed temporal processing impairment to demyelination in the auditory nerve. For example, the failure to detect the evoked auditory brain stem responses in these patients has been related to the loss of discharge synchrony secondary to demyelination of the auditory nerve (Kalaydjieva et al., 1998; Starr et al., 1998). Demyelinated nerve fibers have slowed conduction velocities, which vary as a function of the extent of demyelination in each fiber, resulting in disrupted discharge synchrony both within a neuron and across a neural population.

Figure 8–11 presents a phenomenologic model of the disrupted synchronous neural activity and its account for the present psychophysical data. It could be assumed that the main effect of the desynchronous activity is a smeared temporal representation of the acoustic stimulus (see the difference between the sharp waveform in the physical representation and its smeared version in the internal representation). If the listening task was to detect merely either presence (top trace) or absence (bottom trace) of a sound, as in the case of the temporal integration experiment, then this smeared representation would not present a difficult perceptual problem. If the task was to discriminate two different waveforms, however, one with a gap (top trace) and one without gap (bottom trace), then the smearing in the internal representations would result in a much more difficult perceptual task. A quantitative prediction of the psychophysical data is not possible at present and requires much better understanding of the exact physiologic mechanisms of auditory neuropathy (see Harrison, Chapter 4, and Starr, Picton, and Kim, Chapter 5, in this book).

Temporal Processing Deficits

Temporal processing deficits have also been observed in elderly listeners (Gordon-Salant & Fitzgibbons, 1993), patients with multiple sclerosis (Levine, 1993), and children with learning disabilities (Kraus et al., 1996; Merzenich et al., 1996; Tallal & Piercy, 1973; Tallal et al., 1996; Wright et al., 1997). Similar to the present results, those previous studies also found a

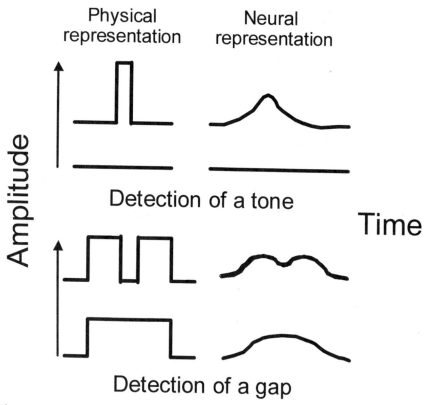

Figure 8–11. A phenomenologic model of auditory neuropathy. This simple model assumes that desynchronous neural activity results in a smeared internal representation of a physical stimulus. The smearing does not affect the detection of a tone (top panel) because the task requires only an all-or-none decision. The smearing can cause a major problem in gap detection (bottom panel) if the task requires finer discrimination of two different waveforms, however.

close relationship between temporal processing and speech recognition deficits, despite a peripheral origin of the temporal processing impairment in auditory neuropathy and a central origin in the other cases. Our study suggests that simple behavioral gap and temporal modulation detection tasks, when used in combination with other audiologic and neurologic tests, can distinguish the extent of temporal processing impairment due to auditory neuropathy in those communication disorders. For example, abnormal temporal processing may reveal the presence of disordered auditory nerve synchrony when there is a concomitant cochlear hearing loss, as occurs in aging.

Other Functional Deficits

We recently have presented preliminary data in simultaneous, forward, and backward masking and found excessive masking for people with AN (Zeng, Oba, & Starr, in press). In particular, we observed abnormally steep growth of masking function for brief tones in noise (2 dB vs. 1 dB) but not for long tones in noise where 1 dB increase in masker level results in 1 dB increase in tone-detection level.

We have not yet systematically studied binaural function in subjects with AN. Previous studies suggested that they could not reliably use binaural temporal cues in interaural timing differences and binaural masking release (Starr et al., 1991). Our study suggests that the difficulty that patients with AN have with binaural tasks may be related to the temporal processing deficits demonstrated in monaural tasks. For example, the smeared temporal representation would impair the ability of patients with AN to perform binaural tasks requiring preservation of precise timing cues. Their significant temporal processing disorder would predict that people with AN should have significant problems in sound localization and in speech recognition under realistic listening situations (e.g., noise and the cocktail party effect).

Reclassification of Hearing Loss

Traditionally, hearing loss has been classified into conductive and sensorineural types, which can be distinguished based on simple tests such as air- versus bone-conduction thresholds. Sensorineural hearing loss can be further classified into cochlear and retrocochlear loss, with the cochlear loss typically demonstrating loudness recruitment and no tone decay. Retrocochlear loss typically refers to the presence of acoustic tumors. Where AN will fall in this classification scheme will depend on further studies isolating the site of lesion. If AN is mainly due to demyelination in the auditory nerve, then it would be best classified into the retrocochlear loss category. If it is mainly due to inner hair cell loss or a dysfunction in the synaptic transduction, then it would be better classified as cochlear loss. Both Starr and Harrison present detailed analysis of both scenarios in this volume. In any case, AN clearly presents a type of hearing loss that is distinct from outer hair cell loss. As we gain additional knowledge about AN, traditional hearing loss classification will have to be modified and refined.

Rehabilitation Strategies

Our results also bear on the failure of conventional hearing aids to help people with AN, who often complain: "I can hear you, but I cannot under-

stand you." Conventional hearing aids either do not change temporal fluctuations of speech sounds (using linear amplification) or even reduce the
fluctuations when a nonlinear amplitude-compression circuit is employed
(Van Tasell, 1993). To improve speech recognition in this population, a new
type of hearing aid design is needed. This design should not only amplify
the sound to overcome the audiometric hearing loss at the threshold level
but also should accentuate temporal envelope fluctuations to compensate
for the impaired temporal processing at suprathreshold levels. For an account of the use of traditional amplification in patients with AN, see Cone-
Wesson, Rance, and Sininger, Chapter 12, in this volume.

In cases of mild to severe neuropathy, hearing aids performing temporal envelope expansion may be enough to compensate for the impaired
temporal processing. Cochlear implants, on the other hand, may be an
effective alternative to treat AN. If the source of this disorder is at the
inner hair cells or synapse, then cochlear implant would be perfect because it bypasses these two stages of processes and directly stimulates
the auditory nerve. In this case, a presurgical promontory stimulation
should be performed to determine whether reliable electrically evoked
potentials can be obtained. Even in the case of neural demyelination or
axonal loss, the cochlear implant may be more effective than the hearing
aid because electrical stimulation has been known to produce more synchronized neural activities than any acoustic stimulation (Dynes and Delgutte, 1992). Clearly, more research is needed to better diagnose and treat
people with AN.

SUMMARY

Our data show that people with AN uniformly have a deficit in temporal
processing and poor frequency discrimination at low and moderate frequencies while having relatively normal intensity processing and normal
frequency discrimination at high frequencies. Correlation analysis suggests that the severe impairment in temporal processing is likely the major
factor contributing to poor speech recognition in people with this disorder.
This conclusion is further supported by a simulation of this temporal processing impairment, which produce similar speech recognition deficits in
listeners with normal hearing. Our data not only demonstrate the importance of neural synchrony for auditory perception, but also provide guidance for better diagnosis and treatment of auditory neuropathy.

Acknowledgments: This work was supported by National Institutes of Health
Grant No. DC02267 and Grant No. DC02618. We thank Chuck Berlin for help in
recruiting subjects and all participants in the experiments for their enthusiasm and

persistence. Sid Bacon, Craig Formby, Sandy Gordon-Salant, and Neal Viemeister provided helpful comments on an earlier version of the manuscript.

REFERENCES

Allen, J. B., Hall, J. L., & Jeng, P. S. (1990). Loudness growth in ½-octave bands (LGOB)—A procedure for the assessment of loudness. *Journal of the Acoustical Society of America, 88,* 745–753.

Arai, T., & Greenberg, S. (1998). Speech intelligibility in the presence of cross-channel spectral asynchrony. *Proceedings of the IEEE International Conference on Acoustic Speech Signal Processing,* 933–936.

Bacon, S. P., & Gleitman, R. M. (1992). Modulation detection in subjects with relatively flat hearing losses. *Journal of Speech and Hearing Research, 35,* 642–653.

Bacon, S. P., & Viemeister, N. F. (1985). Temporal modulation transfer functions in normal-hearing and hearing-impaired listeners. *Audiology, 24,* 117–134.

Drullman, R., Festen, J. M., & Plomp, R. (1994). Effect of temporal envelope smearing on speech reception. *Journal of the Acoustical Society of America, 95,* 1053–1064.

Dubno, J. R., & Ahlstrom, J. B. (1995). Masked thresholds and consonant recognition in low-pass maskers for hearing-impaired and normal-hearing listeners. *Journal of the Acoustical Society of America, 97,* 2430–2441.

Dynes, S. B., & Delgutte, B. (1992). Phase-locking of auditory-nerve discharges to sinusoidal electric stimulation of the cochlea. *Hearing Research, 58,* 79–90.

Fitzgibbons, P. J., & Gordon-Salant, S. (1987). Minimum stimulus levels for temporal gap resolution in listeners with sensorineural hearing loss. *Journal of the Acoustical Society of America, 81,* 1542–1545.

Florentine, M., & Buus, S. (1984). Temporal gap detection in sensorineural and simulated hearing impairments. *Journal of Speech and Hearing Research, 27,* 449–455.

Formby, C., & Muir, K. (1988). Modulation and gap detection for broadband and filtered noise signals. *Journal of the Acoustical Society of America, 84,* 545–550.

Gordon-Salant, S., & Fitzgibbons, P. J. (1993). Temporal factors and speech recognition performance in young and elderly listeners. *Journal of Speech and Hearing Research, 36,* 1276–1285.

Greenberg, S., & Arai, T. (1998). Speech intelligibility is highly tolerant of cross-channel spectral asynchrony. *Proceedings of the Joint Meeting of the Acoustical Society of America and the International Congress on Acoustics, 4,* 2677–2678.

Harrison, R. V. (1998). An animal model of auditory neuropathy. *Ear and Hearing, 19,* 355–361.

Hellman, R. P., & Zwislocki, J. J. (1963). Monaural loudness function at 1000 cps and interaural summation. *Journal of the Acoustical Society of America, 35,* 856–865.

Kalaydjieva, L., Nikolova, A., Turnev, I., Petrova, J., Hristova, A., Ishpekova, B., Petkova, I., Shmarov, A., Stancheva, S. Middleton, L., Merlini, L., Trogu, A., Muddle, J. R., King, R. H., & Thomas, P. K. (1998). Hereditary motor and sensory neuropathy-Lom, a novel demyelinating neuropathy associated with deafness in Gypsies. Clinical, electrophysiological and nerve biopsy findings. *Brain, 121,* 399–408.

Kraus, N., McGee, T. J., Carrell, T. D., Zecker, S. G., Nicol, T. G., & Koch, D. B. (1996). Auditory neurophysiologic responses and discrimination deficits in children with learning problems. *Science, 273,* 971–973.

Levine, R. A. (1993). Effects of multiple sclerosis brainstem lesions on sound lateralization and brainstem auditory evoked potentials. *Hearing Research, 68,* 73–88.

Merzenich, M. M., Jenkins, W. M., Johnston, P., Schreiner, C., Miller, S. L., & Tallal, P. (1996). Temporal processing deficits of language-learning impaired children ameliorated by training. *Science, 271,* 77–81.

Moore, B. C. J., & Glasberg, B. R. (1988). Gap detection with sinusoids and noise in normal, impaired and electrically stimulated ears. *Journal of the Acoustical Society of America, 83,* 1093–1101.

Moore, B. C. J., Shailer, M. J., & Schooneveldt, G. P. (1992). Temporal modulation transfer functions for band-limited noise in subjects with cochlear hearing loss. *British Journal of Audiology, 26,* 229–237.

Mueller, H. G., & Killion, M. C. (1990). An easy method for calculating the Articulation Index. *Hearing Journal 43,* 14–17.

Shannon, R. V., Zeng, F. G., Wygonski, J., Kamath, V., & Ekelid, M. (1995). Speech recognition with primarily temporal cues. *Science, 270,* 303–304.

Starr, A., McPherson, D., Patterson, J., Don, M., Luxford, W., Shannon, R., Sininger, Y., Tonakawa, L., & Waring, M. (1991) Absence of both auditory evoked potentials and auditory percepts dependent on timing cues. *Brain, 114,* 1157–1180.

Starr, A., Picton, T. W., Sininger, Y., Hood, L. J., & Berlin, C. I. (1996). Auditory neuropathy. *Brain, 119,* 741–753.

Starr, A., Sininger, Y., Winter, M., Derebery, M. J., Oba, S., & Michalewski, H. J. (1998). Transient deafness due to temperature-sensitive auditory neuropathy. *Ear and Hearing, 19,* 169–179.

Tallal, P., Miller, S. L., Bedi, G., Byma, G., Wang, X., Nagarajan, S. S., Schreiner, C., Jenkins, W. M., & Merzenich, M. M. (1996). Language comprehension in language-learning impaired children improved with acoustically modified speech. *Science, 271,* 81–84.

Tallal, P., & Piercy, M. (1973). Defects of non-verbal auditory perception in children with developmental aphasia. *Nature, 241,* 468–469.

Van Tasell, D. J. (1993). Hearing loss, speech, and hearing aids. *Journal of Speech and Hearing Research, 36,* 228–244.

Van Tasell, D. J., Soli, S. D., Kirby, V. M., & Widin, G. P. (1987). Speech waveform envelope cues for consonant recognition. *Journal of the Acoustical Society of America, 82,* 1152–1161.

Viemeister, N. F. (1979). Temporal modulation transfer functions based upon modulation thresholds. *Journal of the Acoustical Society of America, 66,* 1364–1380.

Wright, B. A., Lombardino, L. J., King, W. M., Puranik, C. S., Leonard, C. M., & Merzenich, M. M. (1997). Deficits in auditory temporal and spectral resolution in language-impaired children. *Nature, 387,* 176–178.

Zeng, F. G., Oba, S., Garde, S., Sininger, Y., & Starr, A. (1999). Temporal and speech processing deficits in auditory neuropathy. *NeuroReport, 10,* 3429–3435.

Zeng, F. G., Oba, S., & Starr, A. (in press). Suprathreshold processing deficits due to desynchrounous neural activities in auditory neuropathy. In A. J. M. Houtsma, A. Kohlrausch, V. F. Prijs, R. Schoonhoven (Eds.), *Physiological and psychophysical bases of auditory function.* Maastricht, Netherlands: Shaker Publishing BV.

Zwislocki, J. J. (1965). Analysis of some auditory characteristics. In R. D. Luce et al. (Eds.), *Handbook of mathematical psychology* (pp. 80–96). New York: John Wiley.

9

The Genetics
of Auditory Neuropathy

*Renee Rogers, William J. Kimberling, Arnold Starr,
Karin Kirschhofer, Edward Cohn, Judith B. Kenyon,
and Bronya J. Keats*

Auditory neuropathies are a clinically and genetically heterogeneous set of hearing disorders in which neural function is impaired, but the outer hair cells of the cochlea appear to function normally. Most cases are sporadic, but families with two or more affected individuals have been described. In some of these families affected individuals have an affected parent, which suggests an autosomal dominant pattern of inheritance, and affected members of these families often present with a peripheral neuropathy resembling Charcot-Marie-Tooth disease. The hearing problems tend to begin with difficulty understanding what is being said when there is background noise and may progress to severe hearing loss (Hamiel et al., 1993; Musiek, Weider, & Mueller, 1982; Raglan, Prasher, Trinder, & Rudge, 1987). In other families, the parents are not affected but they have two or more offspring with auditory neuropathy, a pattern that is consistent with autosomal recessive inheritance. Infants with autosomal recessive forms of auditory neuropathy often present with profound hearing impairment. Although their auditory brain stem responses (ABRs) and middle ear muscle reflexes are absent, these patients have robust otoacoustic emissions (OAEs; Berlin et al., 1998; Starr, Picton, Sininger, Hood, & Berlin, 1996). An alternative presentation is an audiogram showing a range of hearing levels that span from normal hearing or mild-to-moderate hearing impairment, but absent or abnormal ABR results, poor speech discrimination, and great difficulty hearing in noise (Kraus, Ozdamar, Stein, & Reed, 1984; Kraus et al., 1993; Starr et al., 1991; Worthington & Peters, 1980). Associated peripheral neuropathy is usually not found with autosomal recessive auditory neuropathy. An exception is a Roma family in which affected members have hereditary sensory motor neuropathy and neural deafness (Kalaydjieva et al., 1996, 1998).

Many families with auditory neuropathy have been identified, but the location of the gene responsible for the pathology has been determined in only one. The difficulties with finding these genes are the small sizes of the families and the high level of heterogeneity, with many different genes resulting in similar phenotypes. Additionally, in some children diagnosed with an auditory neuropathy, OAEs disappear faster than expected as they get older. Thus, diagnosing the disorder in older children may be problematic. The gene localized in the large Roma kindred is on the long arm of chromosome 8 (Kalaydjieva et al., 1996). The disorder is recessive in this kindred, but because of the isolated and endogamous nature of the Roma population, 14 affected individuals spanning four generations participated in the study. OAEs were not obtained on these patients; however, Butinar et al. (1999) performed extensive auditory testing on members of another Roma family with a similar phenotype, showing linkage to the same region of chromosome 8. The affected members in this family had abnormal ABRs but robust OAEs, indicating auditory neuropathy.

THE HUMAN GENOME

Each person has two sets of 23 chromosomes. One is the paternal set (inherited from the father), and the other is the maternal set (inherited from the mother). This makes a total of 46 chromosomes in each cell, except in the sex cells or gametes (eggs for female and sperm for male). The sex cells undergo a process called meiosis so that they contain only one copy of each chromosome. When they fuse during conception, the resulting cell, the fertilized egg, will have the 46 chromosomes required to make a new human being.

Each chromosome contains many genes, which carry the "blueprint" for each living thing. The estimated 80,000 to 120,000 pairs of human genes carry the necessary information to cause a single cell, the fertilized egg, to grow into a human being.

GENETIC HEARING LOSS

It is estimated that in at least half of all cases of childhood hearing loss, the etiology is genetic. About one quarter of the cases of childhood hearing loss result from nongenetic causes, and the cause of the remaining 25% is unknown. It is reasonable to suspect that at least half of the "cause un-

Hearing Loss Etiologies

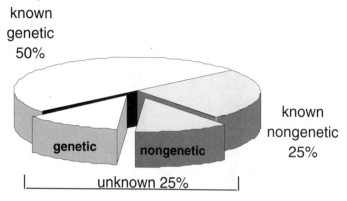

Figure 9–1. This pie graph shows the distribution of the causes of hearing loss.

known" cases are also genetic (Figure 9–1). If that is true, more than 60% of childhood hearing loss is hereditary.

Studies indicate that about 80% of those with hereditary hearing loss have recessive nonsyndromic deafness (RNSD; Cohn et al., 1999; Morell et al., 1998). Nonsyndromic indicates that there are no additional medical conditions associated with the hearing loss (e.g., in Pendred syndrome, a goiter is associated with the hearing loss). Recessive means that a person must have two copies of a gene (a pair) to have hearing impairment. Individuals with only one RNSD gene do not have a hearing loss, but they are carriers of RNSD. Most carriers do not know they carry the mutated gene. If both members of a couple are carriers of RNSD, then with each pregnancy they have a 25% chance of having a child with RNSD. If the child receives the mutated gene from each parent, that child will have two copies of the mutated gene and will have RNSD (Figure 9–2). Thus, a child may have a hearing loss, but that child's mother, father, grandparents, aunts, and uncles may all have normal hearing for their ages. If a person who has RNSD marries a person who is not a carrier, none of their children will have RNSD; however, all of their children will be carriers. If a person who carries RNSD marries a person who is not a carrier, none of their children will have RNSD, but there is a one in two chance for each child to be a carrier. If two people with RNSD (caused by the same gene) marry, all of their children will have RNSD. The most common type of RNSD is due to mutations in the gene called Connexin 26 (Cx26). OAEs are absent in individuals whose deafness is due to Cx26 mutations (Cohn et al., 1999).

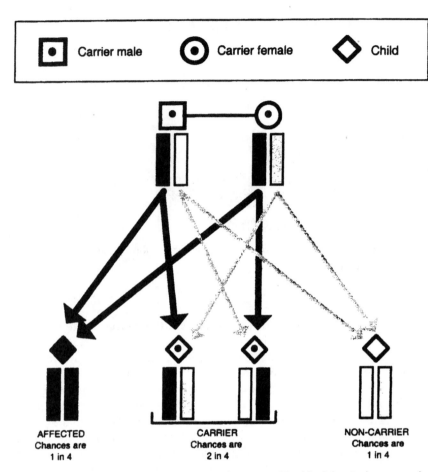

Figure 9–2. This diagram shows recessive inheritance. The black bar is the mutated gene, and the white and shaded bars are the normal copies of the gene.

Recessive auditory neuropathy may present as RNSD that can be differentiated from other cases because of the presence of OAEs.

MATERIALS AND METHODS

To find the gene(s) that causes auditory neuropathy, we draw a small amount of blood from individuals in a family with at least one member affected with auditory neuropathy. The DNA is extracted from the white blood cells in each person's blood sample. We then perform linkage analysis using their DNA to localize the gene to a small region on a specific chromosome.

A linkage study consists of analyzing genetic markers to find one that is close to the auditory neuropathy gene. Markers are short sequences of DNA that vary between individuals, which have been mapped to specific regions in the genome. We must have DNA from at least one affected person and that person's sibling to compare their DNA. If a marker is close to the disease-causing auditory neuropathy gene, affected siblings will have inherited the same marker DNA sequences (alleles) and at least one different allele than that inherited by their unaffected siblings.

If a marker is on the same chromosome as the auditory neuropathy gene but not very close to it, a crossover may occur between the marker and the gene. Crossovers are useful for refining the region containing the gene. The result of a single crossover event for a pair of chromosomes is shown in Figure 9–3. Such an event in the father (I-1) in Figure 9–4 gives rise to the offspring II-1. Double crossing over may also take place as is seen in II-2, who is a maternal double crossover. In this family, II-1 and II-2 have a recessive disease, and they inherited the 2 allele for marker 2 from both parents. Neither of the unaffected children inherited two copies of the 2 allele. These results are consistent with the disease gene being close to marker 2. The positions of the crossovers suggest that marker 1 and marker 3 flank the disease gene. (If the disease gene was close to marker 1, we would not expect any of the children to be affected. If it was close to marker 3, only II-1 should be affected.) In other words, the gene could not be located at the bottom or top of the chromosome because the two affected children have different alleles in those locations and therefore received different forms of the genes that are found in those regions of the chromosome.

These results may occur by chance, however, and the disease gene may not be close to any of these markers; thus, we must perform

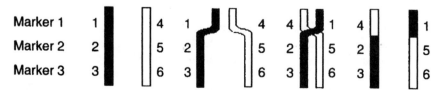

Black = paternal chromosome 1,
White = maternal chromosome 1.
Numbers = allele of the marker

Marker 1	1	4	1	4	4	1	4	1
Marker 2	2	5	2	5	2	5	2	5
Marker 3	3	6	3	6	3	6	3	6

Figure 9–3. This figure shows a single crossover event and how it affects inheritance.

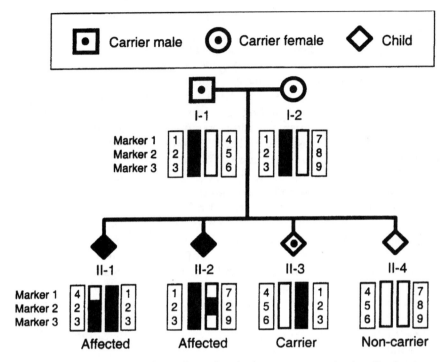

Figure 9–4. This diagram shows how the deafness gene can be localized using haplotyping.

calculations to determine whether this suggestion of linkage is the result of chance. This is done by comparing the likelihood (or probability) that two loci are linked at a given recombination frequency (or fraction) versus the likelihood that the two loci are not linked. The recombination frequency, denoted as θ, is the probability of crossing over between two markers. The recombination frequency can vary between 0, for completely linked loci, and 0.5, for unlinked loci.

For example, suppose we wish to compare the hypothesis that a marker is linked to the disease locus (or gene) at a recombination frequency of $\theta = 0$ versus the hypothesis that the two are not linked. We would form a likelihood ratio:

$$\frac{\text{likelihood of observing pedigree data if } \theta = 0}{\text{likelihood of observing pedigree data if } \theta = 0.5}$$

If the pedigree data indicate that θ is more likely to be 0 than 0.5, then the likelihood ratio will be greater than 1. If the pedigree data argue against linkage of the two loci, then the denominator will be greater than the numerator, and the ratio will be less than 1. The logarithm of the likelihood ratio is denoted as $Z(\theta)$ and called the LOD score. A LOD score of 3 is accepted as evidence of linkage. A LOD score of –2 is accepted as evidence that the two loci are not linked.

Linkage analysis can also be performed with more than two loci. Multipoint analysis uses the same concepts as two point linkage analysis, but the recombination frequencies among all of the loci may be estimated simultaneously.

We have observed three families with two or more children who each have sensorineural hearing loss with normal OAEs (Figure 9–5). All seven individuals with hearing loss, even with normal tympanometry, had absent acoustic reflexes. Degree of hearing loss was determined by a standard pure-tone hearing test. The scale used to classify the degree of hearing loss is as follows: 0–20 dB HL is normal, 21–40 dB HL is mild, 41–60 dB HL is moderate, 61–80 dB HL is severe, and above 80 dB HL is profound. ABR tests were also done to determine the status of the auditory nerve and brain stem pathways. These measurements also were used

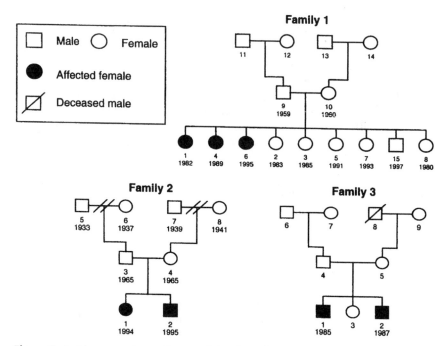

Figure 9–5. These are the pedigrees of the three families studied. The double digit number below the pedigree symbols refers to an identification number of that person. The four-digit number is the year of birth.

to record cochlear microphonics and thus provide another test of hair cell function, supplementing the information provided by the OAE tests. All individuals diagnosed with hearing loss were examined by an ear, nose, and throat (ENT) physician and a geneticist. Tests were performed to rule out symptoms indicating other syndromic disorders. Tests included neurologic exam, eye exam, vestibular ocular reflex (VOR or rotary chair), bithermal calorics, CT (computerized axial tomography), ECG (electrocardiogram), perchlorate discharge, and urinalysis. Cochlear microphonics (CM), distortion-product OAE (DPOAE; Kemp, 1978), or transient-evoked OAE (TEOAE; Martin, Probst, & Lonsbury-Martin, 1990) were used to measure outer hair cell function.

It was determined that the hearing losses of all the affected children were not caused by a known syndrome. According to their families, to speech reception threshold (SRT) testing, or both, these children received no benefit from hearing aids and have speech comprehension loss that is out of proportion to their pure-tone audiograms. The clinical details of all the affected children are summarized in Table 9–1.

Family 1 Clinical Details

Family 1, in Figure 9–5, of European ancestry, has 9 children, 3 of whom have sensorineural hearing loss. There is no other family history of hearing loss. The father, who was tested at Boys Town in 1982 and 1997, had borderline normal hearing. The mother was tested at the same times and had normal hearing.

The youngest affected child in Family 1 (Individual 6), born in 1995, has severe-to-profound sensorineural hearing loss. DPOAEs were present at 2000 to 8000 Hz bilaterally. The ENT exam, eye exam, urinalysis and ECG were all normal. The CT indicated a mild prominence of the vestibules bilaterally (which might be a normal variant) and a minimal amount of fluid in the mastoid air cells bilaterally. Because the patient could not lie still for coronal imaging, the CT was considered incomplete. No dysmorphic features were noted by the geneticist. The rotary chair indicated normal vestibular function in at least one ear. The neurologic exam was normal, and there was no evidence of peripheral neuropathy. Click-evoked ABR testing done at 1 month of age showed no response at 90 dB bilaterally.

Individual 4, born in 1989, has a severe sensorineural hearing loss. In May 1997, DPOAEs were present at 4000–8000 Hz in the right ear and absent in the left ear. A head CT was performed in January 1990 because her skull had a rather unusual shape, which suggested craniosynostosis. The results from the CT scan suggested mild cerebral atrophy. No definite area of suture closure was noticed, however. No gross abnormality was identified in the middle or inner ears bilaterally, and the internal auditory

Table 9–1. Clinical details of the affected children in each of the families.

Individuals	ABR	CM	OAE	Acoustic Reflexes	ENT Exam	Neurologic Exam
			Tests			
Family 1 Ind. 6	absent bilat.	could not be defined	bilat. +	absent	normal	normal
Family 1 Ind. 4	absent bilat.	could not be defined	R +4–8 kHz	absent	normal	normal
Family 1 Ind. 1	absent bilat.	bilat. +	R +6 kHz L absent	absent	normal	normal
Family 2 Ind. 2	absent bilat.	bilat. +	bilat. +	absent	normal	normal
Family 2 Ind. 1	absent bilat.	bilat. +	bilat. +	absent	normal	normal
Family 3 Ind. 2	absent bilat.	R + L DNT	bilat. +	absent	normal	normal
Family 3 Ind. 1	absent bilat.	bilat. +	bilat. +	absent	normal	normal

Note. ABR = auditory brain stem response test; CM = cochlear microphonics; ENT exam = ear, nose, throat physician's exam; DNT = did not test; + = present; bilat. = bilaterally; R = right; L = left; Ind. = Individual.

canals were normal. At 9 months of age, skull X-rays were taken that demonstrated that the overall appearance of the skull was within normal limits. The ENT exam, eye exam, ECG, urinalysis, and temporal CT were all normal, and no dysmorphic features were noticed during the geneticist's examination. The rotary chair indicated normal peripheral vestibular function. The neurologic exam was normal. No waveforms were detected bilaterally at the maximum intensity limits of the equipment (95 dB) when clicks were presented with alternating polarity at 2 weeks of age for the ABR test.

The oldest child affected with hearing loss, individual Number 1, was born in 1982. She has a bowl-shaped, severe-to-profound sensorineural hearing loss. The hearing loss was first noted at 7 months of age. In May 1997, speech awareness thresholds (SATs) were consistent with the hearing loss, but SRTs could not be completed because she could not be familiarized to the words at equipment limits. DPOAEs were absent bilaterally except at 6000 Hz in the right ear. The ENT exam, eye exam, ECG, and temporal CT were all normal. The urinalysis was normal in 1982 and normal except for 1+ protein in 1997. No dysmorphic features were noticed by the geneticist. Rotary chair and bithermal caloric responses indicated normal peripheral vestibular function in both ears. The neurologic exam and nerve conduction velocities were normal. An ABR, done in 1982, found no replicable responses with stimulation of rarefaction or condensation clicks up to 102 dB, bilaterally. CMs appeared to be present on the left but not on the right. In 1998, CMs were present bilaterally with high-intensity stimulation.

Figure 9–6 shows the audiograms and the DPOAEgrams of the three affected children from Family 1, all taken in May 1997. The audiograms are on top and the DPOAEgrams are on the bottom. The order, from left to right, is youngest to oldest.

Family 2 Clinical Details

Family 2 (see Figure 9–5) is also of European ancestry with no history of hearing loss. This family has two children with profound, bilateral sensorineural hearing loss.

The younger child in this family, Individual 2, was born in 1995 and has profound sensorineural hearing loss. DPOAEs were present for both ears at 1600–4000 Hz. The ENT exam and neurologic exam, which measured peripheral motor and sensory nerve conduction, were normal. No dysmorphic features were noted during the geneticist's exam. The click-evoked ABR done in September 1995 was difficult to interpret but definitely abnormal and consistent with a neuropathy. It indicated a poorly formed wave I and possible wave II deformity bilaterally. We were unable to tell if CMs are present although testing was performed using separate rarefaction and condensation clicks at 95 dB. In contrast, the click-evoked ABR from June 1998 showed absent neural components, as well as both CM and transient summating potential (SP) bilaterally. The SP was revealed when the CMs were attenuated by subtracting condensation–rarefaction traces peaking at a latency of 1.3–1.48 ms. The presence of both CM and SP indicates preserved outer and inner hair cell functions.

Individual 1, born in 1994, also has profound sensorineural hearing loss. TEOAEs were present bilaterally. She had normal ENT, eye, and neurologic exams. The neurologic exam measured peripheral motor and sensory nerve conduction. Results from the rotary chair suggests that peripheral vestibular function is normal. The geneticist's exam was normal, and no dysmorphic features were noted. Magnetic resonance imaging (MRI) showed normal appearing brain and brain stem. The results of an ABR at 15 months indicated only wave I present in the right ear and a possible wave I present in the left ear. Because only rarefaction clicks were used, we are unable to determine if CMs are present. An ABR was also performed at 17 months of age using a tone, rarefaction, and condensation clicks. In the left ear, an 85 dB click and low frequency tone did not elicit

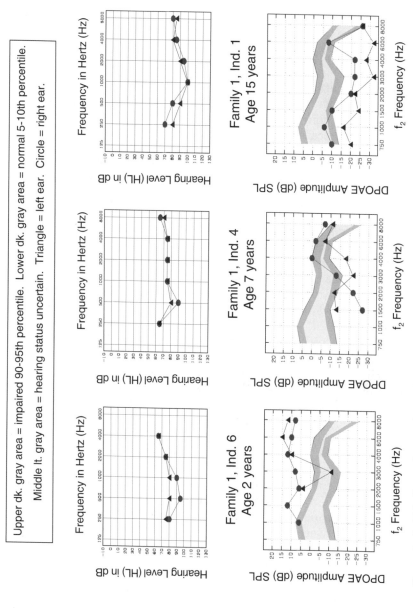

Figure 9–6. This figure depicts the audiograms and DPOAEgrams of the three affected children from Family 1. The results suggest a progressive loss of OHC function with age.

any recognizable waveforms. An 80 dB click did not evoke a response in the right ear. CM is present in the right ear, but the presence of a CM for the left ear cannot be determined. The June 1998 click-evoked ABR showed bilateral absent neural components (waves 1 through V). CM and SP were both present bilaterally.

Family 3 Clinical Details

Family 3 in Figure 9–5 is Native American with two children with sensorineural hearing loss. Other than the father's half-sister's son, who is reported to have a congenital hearing loss and cleft lip/palate, there is no family history of hearing loss.

Individual 2, who was born in 1987, has a gradually sloping severe-to-profound sensorineural hearing loss. He had spinal meningitis, diagnosed by spinal tap, at 10 months of age, after which a click-evoked ABR indicated a severe-to-profound hearing loss. His meningitis was reportedly caused by a virus. The geneticist concluded that the hearing loss is not related to meningitis because there is another affected sibling. In addition, it has been reported that viral meningitis is not often seen to cause hearing loss (Fleischer, 1987; Nadol, 1978; Wilfert et al., 1981). TEOAEs were present bilaterally when tested in November of 1996 and July of 1998. Testing in November 1996 also found present DPOAEs bilaterally. Speech awareness threshold (SAT) at this time was at 70 dB HL in the right ear and at 65 dB HL in the left ear, which were in close agreement with tonal findings. Speech reception threshold (SRT) was attempted but had to be discontinued because he could not be familiarized to the words at 115 dB HL, even when given visual cues. The ENT exam was normal. Between 2 and 3 years of age, he had several fainting spells. There is a maternal family history of fainting spells and migraine headaches. Because of this, several electroencephalograms (EEGs) were done. The EEGs done in January 1990 and July 1995 were normal, but the August 1990 EEG was possibly abnormal. A normal CT scan was reported in 1989. The neurologic exam performed in July 1998, which included peroneal motor nerve conduction and sural nerve conduction, was normal. Rotary chair testing done in November 1996 indicated normal peripheral vestibular function in at least one ear, but also a possible slight asymmetry in vestibular function between ears. The family had not noticed any vestibular problems. Dysmorphic features noted by the medical geneticist were three small linear creases in the backs of the earlobes bilaterally, posterior hair whorl, two pits behind the right ear, and three pits behind the left ear. In July 1998, a click-evoked ABR was performed in the right ear. This revealed an absence of all components beginning with wave I, but CMs were present.

Individual Number 1, the oldest child in the family, was born in 1985. He has a bowl-shaped, moderate-to-severe sensorineural hearing loss. Bilateral normal TEOAEs and DPOAEs were obtained in November 1996 and July 1998. SAT was 45 dB HL bilaterally in November 1996, which is in good agreement with tonal findings; however, SRT results were inconsistent with tonal findings in that testing could not be completed because he was unable to identify spondee pictures consistently at levels of 85 and 105 dB. The ECG, ENT, and eye exams were normal except for slight hyperopia. A neurologic exam was performed in February 1995 because of a history of severe migraine headaches that included dizziness and photophobia. The exam was normal. The neurologic exam performed in July 1998, which included peroneal motor nerve conduction and sural nerve conduction, was also normal. In November 1996, results for the rotary chair suggested normal vestibular function in at least one ear. An MRI was normal with normal-appearing internal auditory canals. Neural responses were absent, but CMs were obtained bilaterally for click-evoked ABRs performed on November 1996 and July 1998. Other than a midline hair whorl, the geneticist noted no dysmorphic features.

DNA Extraction

Blood samples were collected from all informative family members. DNA was extracted using Puregene DNA isolation kits by Gentra Systems. The genomic DNA was PCR (polymerase chain reaction) amplified and genotyped using ABI Prism set 1 dinucleotide markers on an ABI 377 genotyper according to standard protocol (Reed et al., 1994). GeneScan 2.1 and Genotyper 2.0 software were used to analyze gel data. Families were haplotyped and linkage analysis was performed using LINKAGE program version 5.1 (Lathrop, Lalouel, Julier, & Ott, 1984). LOD scores were generated using LINKMAP for multipoint analysis.

RESULTS

Seven children with moderate to profound sensorineural hearing loss from three families were found to have auditory neuropathy. No peripheral neuropathies were observed in any of the children. Their hearing loss, determined by a standard pure-tone hearing test, was not caused by a syndrome or any known nongenetic factors. ABR testing revealed impaired neural function, but the outer hair cells of these children were found to function normally, as determined by OAE and CM testing. The middle ear muscle reflexes were absent even though tympanometry was normal. All the children reported no benefit from hearing aids and had speech comprehension loss that is worse than would be expected by looking at their pure-tone audiograms alone.

Using linkage analysis we found two regions, one on chromosome 1 and one on chromosome 7, that are possible locations for the auditory neuropathy gene. Because of critical crossovers in Families 1 and 2, the gene has been localized on chromosome 1 to the region between D1S209 and D1S207 (Figure 9–7). The region on chromosome 7 is between D7S2444 and D7S484 because of two critical crossovers that occurred in Family 1 (Figure 9–8).

LODs were generated and plotted for 344 markers that spanned the entire genome, except the sex chromosomes, at an average distance of 10 cM (centiMorgans). For Family 1, the only areas compatible with linkage were regions on chromosomes 1, 7, and 21. Family 3 excluded chromosome 21 as a linkage-compatible region. Therefore, this genome scan excluded all areas, except for the critical regions on chromosomes 1 and 7, as being compatible for linkage. Results of the multipoint analysis are consistent with the haplotype data. The highest LOD score on chromosome 1 was 2.905 for marker D1S430. On chromosome 7, the highest LOD score was 2.908 for marker D7S516.

These results strongly indicate that the gene(s) for auditory neuropathy is located in either or both of these two places. It is possible that this is a double recessive trait and that mutations in two different genes need to be inherited together to cause auditory neuropathy.

DISCUSSION

When looking at the audiogram data and DPOAEgram data for Family 1, we noticed that although the audiograms show about the same hearing levels, the DPOAEgrams show that the OAEs seem to deteriorate with age (see Figure 9–6). The youngest, 2 years old, has profound hearing loss and robust OAEs bilaterally. The 7-year-old child has severe hearing loss and absent OAEs except at 4000 to 8000 Hz in the right ear. The 15-year-old child has profound hearing loss and absent OAEs except at 6000 Hz in the right ear. If OAE loss is progressive in auditory neuropathy, then it is possible that adults with auditory neuropathy could be difficult to distinguish from the other nonsyndromic recessive hearing disorders, which are more common than auditory neuropathy, and the frequency of this disorder is greater than previously estimated.

It is possible to localize genetic disorders such as auditory neuropathy by linkage analysis, but it is a long and laborious process because of the size of the human genome. Because auditory neuropathy is rare, it is difficult to find families in the general population, and those that are found are often small, which diminishes the number of informative meioses. As of now there is no way to test clinically for carriers of this recessive disorder, and the amount of information that can be extracted from each sibship is limited because of a lack of phase information between the marker and the disease gene. If OAE responses decrease with age, as they seem to in

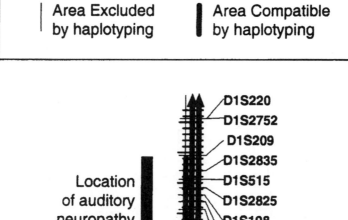

Area Excluded by haplotyping	Area Compatible by haplotyping

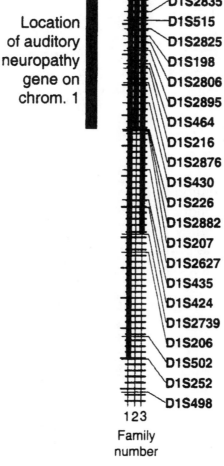

Location of auditory neuropathy gene on chrom. 1

D1S220
D1S2752
D1S209
D1S2835
D1S515
D1S2825
D1S198
D1S2806
D1S2895
D1S464
D1S216
D1S2876
D1S430
D1S226
D1S2882
D1S207
D1S2627
D1S435
D1S424
D1S2739
D1S206
D1S502
D1S252
D1S498

1 2 3

Family number

Figure 9–7. This diagram shows the critical region found on chromosome 1 by haplotyping the three families and the markers used in this area.

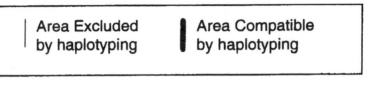

Area Excluded
by haplotyping

Area Compatible
by haplotyping

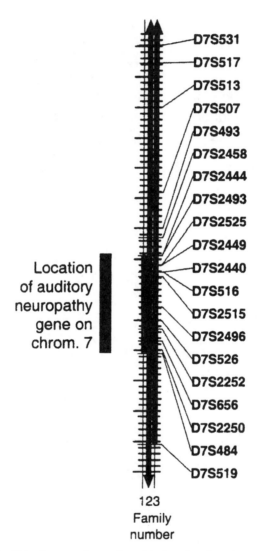

D7S531
D7S517
D7S513
D7S507
D7S493
D7S2458
D7S2444
D7S2493
D7S2525
D7S2449
D7S2440
D7S516
D7S2515
D7S2496
D7S526
D7S2252
D7S656
D7S2250
D7S484
D7S519

Location
of auditory
neuropathy
gene on
chrom. 7

1 2 3
Family
number

Figure 9–8. This diagram shows the critical region found on chromosome 7 by haplotyping the three families and the markers used in this area.

Family 1, then it is more difficult to find families with this condition by clinical means once they have reached an age where the OAE responses have diminished to levels consistent with other hearing losses.

Our ultimate goal is to find and characterize the gene(s) so that a treatment for auditory neuropathy may be developed. We need more families so that we can raise the LOD and refine the critical region(s). More families may also define whether this is a double recessive trait or a single gene disorder.

Acknowledgments: Thank you to Michael Gorga and Mary Ava Grossman for their helpful suggestions. We are grateful to the families for their participation in this research. This work was supported by National Institute on Deafness and Other Communication Disorders Grant No. P01 DC01813.

REFERENCES

Berlin, C. I., Bordelon, J., St. John, P., Wilensky, D., Hurley, A., Kluka, E., & Hood, L. J. (1998). Reversing click polarity may uncover auditory neuropathy in infants. *Ear and Hearing, 19,* 37–47.

Butinar, D., Zidar, J., Leonardis, L., Popovic, M., Kalaydjieva, L., Angelicheva, D., Sininger, Y., Keats, B., & Starr, A. (1999). Hereditary auditory, vestibular, motor, and sensory neuropathy in a Slovenian Roma (Gypsy) kindred. *Annals of Neurology, 46,* 36–44.

Cohn, E. S., Kelley, P. M., Fowler, T. W., Gorga, M. P., Lefkowitz, D. M., Kuehn, H. J., Schaefer, G. B., Gobar, L. S., Hahn, F. J., Harris, D. J., & Kimberling, W. J. (1999). Clinical studies of families with hearing loss attributable to mutations in the connexin 26 gene (GJB2/DFNB1). *Pediatrics, 103,* 546–550.

Fleischer, K. (1987). Horschaden nach Meningitis einst und jetzt. *HNO, 35,* 199–202.

Hamiel, O. P., Raas-Rothschild, A., Upadhyaya, M., Frydman, M., Sarova-Pinhas, I., Brand, N., & Passwell, J. H. (1993). Hereditary motor-sensory neuropathy (Charcot-Marie-Tooth disease) with nerve deafness: A new variant. *Journal of Pediatrics, 123,* 431–434.

Kalaydjieva, L., Hallmayer, J., Chandler, D., Savov, A., Nikolova, A., Angelicheva, D., King, R. H., Ishpekova, B., Honeyman, K., Calafell, F., Shmarov, A., Petrova, J., Turnev, I., Hristova, A., Moskov, M., Stancheva, S., Petkova, I., Bittles, A. H., Georgieva, V., Middleton, L., & Thomas, P. K. (1996). Gene mapping in Gypsies identifies a novel demyelinating neuropathy on chromosome 8q24. *Nature Genetics, 14,* 214–217.

Kalaydjieva, L., Nikolova, A., Turnev, I., Petrova, J., Hristova, A., Ishpekova, B., Petkova, I., Shmarov, A., Stancheva, S., Middleton, L., Merlini, L., Trogu, A., Muddle, J. R., King, R. H., & Thomas, P. K. (1998). Hereditary motor and sensory neuropathy—Lom, a novel demyelinating neuropathy associated with deafness in Gypsies. Clinical, electrophysiological and nerve biopsy findings. *Brain, 121,* 399–408.

Kemp, D. T. (1978). Stimulated acoustic emissions from within the human auditory system. *Journal of the Acoustical Society of America, 64,* 1386–1391.

Kraus, N., McGee, T., Ferre, J., Hoeppner, J. A., Carrell, T., Sharma, A., & Nicol, T. (1993). Mismatch negativity in the neurophysiologic/behavioral evaluation of auditory processing deficits: A case study. *Ear and Hearing, 14,* 223–234.

Kraus, N., Ozdamar, O., Stein, L., & Reed, N. (1984). Absent auditory brain stem response: Peripheral hearing loss or brain stem dysfunction? *Laryngoscope, 94,* 400–406.

Lathrop, G. M., Lalouel, J. M., Julier, C., & Ott, J. (1984). Strategies for multilocus linkage analysis in humans. *Proceedings of the National Academy of Sciences U.S.A., 81,* 3443–3446.

Martin, G. K., Probst, R., & Lonsbury-Martin, B. L. (1990). Otoacoustic emissions in human ears: Normative findings. *Ear and Hearing, 11,* 106–120.

Morel, R. J., Kim, H. J., Hood, L. J., Goforth, L., Friderici, K., Fisher, R., Van Camp, G., Berlin, C. I., Oddoux, C., Ostrer, H., Keats, B., & Friedman, T. B. (1998). Mutations in the connexin 26 gene (GJB2) among Ashkenazi Jews with nonsyndromic recessive deafness. *New England Journal of Medicine, 339,* 1500–1505.

Musiek, F. E., Weider, D. J., & Mueller, R. J. (1982). Audiologic findings in Charcot-Marie-Tooth disease. *Archives of Otolaryngology, 108,* 595–599.

Nadol, J. B. J. (1978). Hearing loss as a sequela of meningitis. *Laryngoscope, 88,* 739–755.

Raglan, E., Prasher, D. K., Trinder, E., & Rudge, P. (1987). Auditory function in hereditary motor and sensory neuropathy (Charcot-Marie-Tooth disease). *Acta Otolaryngology (Stockholm), 103,* 50–55.

Reed, P. W., Davies, J. L., Copeman, J. B., Bennett, S. T., Palmer, S. M., Pritchard, L. E., Gough, S. C., Kawaguchi, Y., Cordell, H. J., & Balfour, K. M. (1994). Chromosome-specific microsatellite sets for fluorescence-based, semi-automated genome mapping. *Nature Genetics, 7,* 390–395.

Starr, A., McPherson, D., Patterson, J., Don, M., Luxford, W., Shannon, R., Sininger, Y., Tonakawa, L., & Waring, M. (1991). Absence of both auditory evoked potentials and auditory percepts dependent on timing cues. *Brain, 114,* 1157–1180.

Starr, A., Picton, T. W., Sininger, Y., Hood, L. J., & Berlin, C. I. (1996). Auditory neuropathy. *Brain, 119,* 741–753.

Wilfert, C. M., Thompson, R. J. J., Sunder, T. R., O'Quinn, A., Zeller, J., & Blacharsh, J. (1981). Longitudinal assessment of children with enteroviral meningitis during the first three months of life. *Pediatrics, 67,* 811–815.

Worthington, D. W., & Peters, J. F. (1980). Quantifiable hearing and no ABR: Paradox or error? *Ear and Hearing, 1,* 281–285.

Auditory Neuropathy (Auditory Dys-synchrony) Disables Efferent Suppression of Otoacoustic Emissions

Linda J. Hood and Charles I. Berlin

Auditory neuropathy (more descriptively named auditory dys-synchrony) in infants, children, and adults reveals itself by the presence of otoacoustic emissions, the absence of a synchronous auditory brain stem response (ABR), and the absence of middle ear muscle reflexes (MEMR) despite normal tympanometry. Clinical findings in patients with auditory neuropathy, as described in Chapter 2 of this book (by Sininger & Oba), indicate variable pure-tone thresholds ranging from normal sensitivity to the severe or profound hearing loss range (e.g., Berlin, Hood, Cecola, Jackson, & Szabo, 1993; Berlin, Hood, Hurley, & Wen, 1994; Gorga, Stelmachowicz, Barlow, & Brookhouser, 1995; Kaga et al., 1996; Starr et al., 1991, 1996). Normal outer hair cell function, at least above 1000 Hz, is marked by the presence of otoacoustic emissions (OAEs) and cochlear microphonics (CMs), which are highlighted by comparing averages obtained using positive versus negative polarity clicks (Berlin et al., 1998). Poor neural synchrony is reflected by abnormal ABRs and absent MEMRs even in the presence of mild or no pure-tone hearing loss. Patients generally show no masking-level difference, which is consistent with abnormalities in processing of timing and phase information. Speech recognition is quite variable, although typically much poorer than expected, and is generally poor in noise or with competing messages.

In addition, patients with auditory neuropathy lack efferent suppression of transient-evoked otoacoustic emissions (TEOAEs; Berlin et al., 1994; Hood et al., 2000). This chapter focuses on function of the olivocochlear system and characteristics of efferent suppression of TEOAEs in individuals with normal auditory function and in patients with auditory neuropathy. Suppression effects on TEOAEs are described for binaural, ipsilateral, and contralateral suppressor stimuli.

THE OLIVOCOCHLEAR PATHWAYS

Auditory efferent fibers travel from the olivocochlear bundle at the level of the olivary complex in the brain stem through the vestibulocochlear (8th) nerve to the cochlea (Figure 10–1). The medial olivocochlear (MOC) fibers terminate primarily on the outer hair cells, whereas the lateral olivocochlear fibers terminate mainly on primary auditory neurons at the base of the inner hair cells (Warr & Guinan, 1978; Warr, Guinan, & White, 1986). In Figure 10–1, illustrating the MOC pathways to one cochlea, the contralaterally responsive pathway is shown to involve the uncrossed olivocochlear fibers (UOCB; see Figure 10–1), whereas the ipsilaterally responsive pathway is shown to involve the crossed olivocochlear fibers (COCB; see Figure 10–1). Thus, the ipsilateral pathway involves crossing of both the afferent and efferent fibers, whereas the contralateral pathway involves only crossed afferent fibers.

Outer hair cell activity is believed to be modified through the MOC efferent connections, while the functional effects of the lateral efferent system remain unknown. The origin of OAEs is ascribed to functions associ-

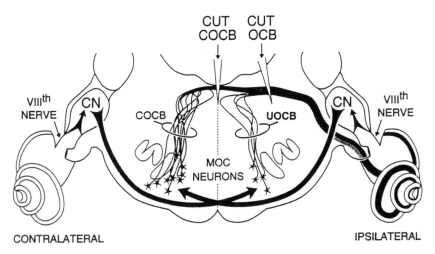

Figure 10–1. Schematic transverse section through the brain stem illustrating the medial olivocochlear pathways in one cochlea. Reprinted with permission from Liberman (1989).

ated with active cochlear processes and the mechanical motion of the outer hair cells. Changes to emissions in the presence of noise are thought to be modulated through the efferent auditory pathways via the olivo-cochlear system (Kemp, 1978; Kemp & Chum, 1980).

OLIVOCOCHLEAR EFFECTS ON OAES AND ACTION POTENTIALS

Function of the medial olivocochlear pathway can be studied objectively and noninvasively in both animals and humans by observing changes in OAEs and compound 8th nerve action potentials. Spontaneous and transient evoked OAEs usually decrease in amplitude with contralateral acoustic stimuli in humans with normal auditory function (Berlin, Hood, Wen et al., 1993; Collet et al., 1990; Grose, 1983; Mott et al., 1989; Rabino-witz & Widen, 1984; Ryan et al., 1991; Schloth & Zwicker, 1983; Veuillet et al., 1991). The effects of contralateral stimuli on distortion product oto-acoustic emissions (DPOAE) appear more variable, with reports of both increases and decreases in DPOAE amplitude with presentation of contra-lateral stimuli (Moulin et al., 1992, 1993; Nieschall et al., 1997; Timpe-Syverson & Decker, 1999). Efferent effects on the compound action potential (ABR wave I) amplitude also have been reported in humans related to suppression (Folsom & Owsley, 1987) and release from masking (Kawase & Takasaka, 1995)

Olivocochlear stimulation effects observed in humans are consistent with observations of suppression of both cochlear emissions and auditory nerve activity in animals. Galambos (1956) first described reduced ampli-tude of the compound action potential with electrical stimulation of the olivocochlear bundle. Later studies confirmed this observation for both OAEs and neural responses (e.g., Brown & Nuttall, 1984; Buno, 1978; Liberman, 1989; Mountain, 1980; Puel & Rebillard, 1990).

CHARACTERISTICS OF SUPPRESSION IN INDIVIDUALS WITH NORMAL AUDITORY FUNCTION

Activation of the efferent system alters OAEs. The effect is generally re-ferred to as suppression, based on the characteristic decrease in OAE amplitude in the presence of a suppressor stimulus. Because OAE sup-pression represents function of a feedback loop or reflex, it is also de-scribed as the olivocochlear reflex or the medial olivocochlear reflex.

Efferent suppression of TEOAEs can be recorded by introducing a suppressor stimulus into the opposite ear, the same ear, or in both ears.

In the contralateral suppression mode, a continuous noise is presented to the opposite ear during the time that the emission is recorded and averaged. This is the most commonly used method to study efferent suppression and perhaps the easiest and most rapid way to study the effect. Nonetheless, binaural suppressor stimuli result in larger suppression effects than contralaterally presented suppressors (Berlin et al., 1995).

When suppression is studied while presenting a suppressor stimulus to the same ear from which the TEOAE is recorded, it is not possible to present the emission-evoking stimulus and the suppressor stimulus simultaneously without producing unwanted interactions between the OAE evoking stimulus and the suppressor stimulus. Therefore, a forward-masking paradigm is employed when studying ipsilateral and binaural suppression effects. For consistency, we also study contralateral effects in a forward-masking paradigm to compare suppression effects among the three modes of suppressor presentation (contralateral, ipsilateral, binaural).

RECORDING AND ANALYZING TEOAE SUPPRESSION

Efferent suppression of TEOAEs is assessed in our laboratory and clinical practice using 55 to 65 dB peak SP (sound pressure) linear clicks and noise levels of 60 to 70 dB SPL (sound pressure level). These stimulus levels are based on studies that demonstrated greater suppression effects for lower rather than higher intensity clicks (Hood et al., 1996; Veuillet et al., 1991). Furthermore, these intensities maximize the suppression effect while minimizing against the use of intensity levels that may evoke a middle ear muscle response. Click stimuli that employ all clicks with the same polarity are recommended to avoid distortions in response amplitude (Berlin et al., 1995; Collet et al., 1990).

We interleave two or three "without noise" and two or three "with noise" conditions, assure that the stimulus intensity remains constant, analyze results using the Kresge Laboratory EchoMaster software (see Appendix), and focus on the 8- to 18-ms time period. Monitoring the suppressor level with a low-noise probe microphone in the ear canal is critical to ensure that an accurate and constant suppressor intensity is maintained throughout testing.

Suppressor stimuli can be tones, narrow band noise, broadband noise, modulated signals, speech, or other types of stimuli that are relatively continuous or long in duration. When using click stimuli to elicit the TEOAE, broadband suppressor stimuli are most effective with narrowband noise and tonal suppressors showing less suppression (Berlin, Hood, Wen et al., 1993). Amplitude- and frequency-modulated stimuli also have been reported to elicit robust efferent suppression responses (Maison et al., 1998).

Most studies of suppression of TEOAEs have used continuous contra-lateral noise (e.g., Berlin, Hood, Wen et al., 1993; Collet et al., 1990; Ryan et al., 1991). To study efferent function more fully and to assess the contra-lateral and ipsilateral pathways in humans, Berlin et al. (1995) applied a forward-masking paradigm, in which the suppressor precedes the test stimulus (i.e., the click or toneburst) used to elicit the TEOAE in time. This allowed us to study the effects of ipsilateral and binaural suppressors as well as contralateral suppressors on TEOAEs. The anatomy predicted the result; noise binaurally presented produces significantly greater suppres-sion than ipsilateral or contralateral noise. Despite being the most com-monly used type of suppression measure, continuous contralateral noise generates the smallest result (Berlin et al., 1995).

We report suppression effects as dB differences in emission amplitude between conditions with and without suppression signals. The observa-tion of greater suppression effects in certain time periods led to the devel-opment of the Kresge EchoMaster method to analyze suppression of emissions in greater detail (Wen et al., 1993).

Figure 10–2 (lower portion) provides an example of TEOAEs obtained with and without continuous contralateral broadband noise. The emission amplitude is plotted as a function of time. By plotting amplitude in 1-, 2-, or 3-ms intervals, it is possible to obtain greater detail and more accu-rate quantification of suppression in various time periods. The root mean square amplitude differences between the TEOAE with and without noise, calculated by the EchoMaster analysis, are shown in the upper portion of Figure 10–2. Note that the maximum amplitude differences between the without noise and with noise conditions are concentrated in the time period between 8 and 18 ms. This region is bracketed by the bars in the lower portion of the figure. Recall that the time domain also represents frequency with shorter latencies depicting higher frequencies and longer latencies for lower frequencies. Time as well as amplitude shifts occur in many individuals, as indicated by the "delay" trace in the upper portion of Figure 10–2.

Describing suppression over the entire 20-ms time window with a single number generally underestimates the suppression effect. A detailed analysis of TEOAEs for changes in amplitude, phase, or both, particularly in the 8- to 18-ms time period, provides greater assurance of correctly identifying the presence or absence of an efferent suppression effect.

CHARACTERISTICS OF SUPPRESSION OF TEOAES IN NORMAL INDIVIDUALS

Using the recording and analysis paradigms described previously, we and others have found that efferent suppression of TEOAEs can be character-ized as follows:

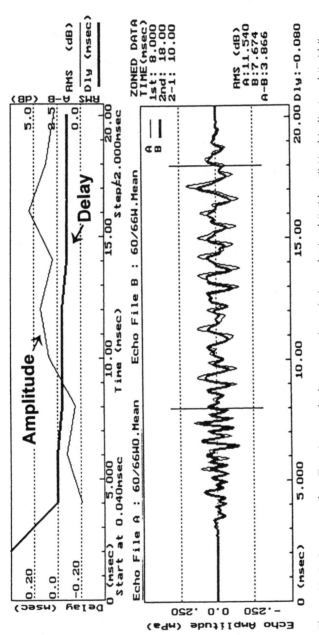

Figure 10–2. Lower portion: Transient-evoked otoacoustic emissions obtained "without" (A, thin line) and "with" suppressor noise (B, thick line) in a normal individual. Emission amplitude in the bracketed region (8–18 ms) is 11.6 dB without noise and 7.7 with noise (binaurally presented). Note the amplitude decreases and shifts in the peaks with noise. **Upper portion:** Quantification of suppression using the Kresge EchoMaster program. Amplitude and time differences between the "without" and "with" suppressor noise conditions in 2-ms intervals are shown for a normal individual.

1. A reduction in amplitude, time changes, or phase shifts of emission peaks, or both (e.g., Berlin, Hood, Cecola et al., 1993; Berlin et al., 1994; Collet et al., 1990; Ryan et al., 1991).
2. Greatest in the 8- to 18-ms time period and in the lower frequencies (e.g., Berlin, Hood, Cecola et al., 1993; Berlin et al., 1994; Collet et al., 1990; Hood et al., 1996; Veuillet et al., 1991).
3. As the intensity of the suppressor noise increases, the amount of suppression increases and the frequency range where suppression is observed broadens.
4. Suppression is proportionately greater for lower intensity stimuli than for higher intensity stimuli (Hood et al., 1996; Ryan & Kemp, 1996; Veuillet et al., 1991).
5. Suppression of TEOAEs is greater for binaural noise than for ipsilateral or contralateral noise and contralateral noise is the least effective suppressor (Berlin et al., 1995).
6. Suppression effects are repeatable both within subjects and between groups (Berlin et al., 1991).

POTENTIAL PROBLEMS AND OTHER CONSIDERATIONS

Middle ear muscle reflexes and acoustic crosstalk or crossover of sound through the head can contaminate measurement of efferent suppression. The occurrence of greater suppression for lower intensity stimuli minimizes the potential role of the middle ear muscle reflex and crossover. If suppression was related to either of these phenomena, then suppression would be expected to increase at higher intensities. In addition, suppression has been observed in patients who lack stapedius muscle function because of either Bell's palsy or stapedius tendon section during stapedectomy. These potential problems underline the importance of monitoring stimulus and suppressor levels during testing.

EFFERENT SUPPRESSION IN PATIENTS WITH AUDITORY NERVE DISORDERS

Patients with auditory neuropathy can be contrasted from those with radiologically or surgically documented space-occupying or other lesions of the 8th nerve based on normal computerized tomography (CT) and magnetic resonance imaging (MRI) results in auditory neuropathy patients. Disruption of suppression of OAEs is observed in both types of disorders.

Many patients with space-occupying 8th nerve lesions demonstrate an absence of OAEs. In those patients where OAEs are present, a lack of efferent suppression is reported in several studies (Liang et al., 1997; Maurer et al., 1992; Prasher et al., 1994). A lack of efferent suppression has been demonstrated in patients who undergo vestibular neurectomy (Giraud et al., 1995; Williams et al., 1993, 1994). This procedure involves sectioning the inferior vestibular fibers, which carry both medial and lateral efferent bundles, with the goal of alleviating vertigo while preserving hearing.

EFFERENT SUPPRESSION IN PATIENTS WITH AUDITORY DYS-SYNCHRONY/NEUROPATHY

Like the patients with space-occupying lesions cited previously, patients with auditory neuropathy consistently show no or minimal suppression of TEOAEs for binaural, ipsilateral, and contralateral suppressor stimuli. Measuring suppression with the detailed EchoMaster analysis method improves the precision in demonstrating either a marked reduction or absence of suppression in these patients. Two case examples of patients with auditory dys-synchrony/neuropathy are presented: one with bilateral and one with unilateral findings. The discussion to follow includes case history, behavioral and physiologic auditory test results, and comparisons of efferent suppression in these patients to suppression in normal individuals.

Case Study 1: Bilateral Auditory Dys-Synchrony/Neuropathy and Abnormal Efferent Suppression of TEOAEs

This female patient has a long-standing hearing loss, first identified in childhood but possibly congenital. There is a positive history of encephalopathy and familial cerebellar syndrome. There is no history of middle ear problems, noise exposure, or ototoxicity. This patient has been followed for many years at Kresge Hearing Research Laboratory and was known to have very poor speech understanding and a dys-synchronous ABR. It was not until OAEs were available that some aspect of normal function at the level of the cochlea was determined. This patient is among those from Kresge Hearing Research Laboratory included in the original group of auditory neuropathy patients described by Berlin et al. (1994) and Starr et al. (1996).

Audiologic pure-tone thresholds, obtained at age 51 years, indicated a bilateral moderately severe hearing loss in the low frequencies rising to thresholds in the normal-to-mild hearing loss range in the higher frequencies (Figure 10–3). Ipsilateral and contralateral middle ear muscle reflexes were absent, despite normal middle ear function.

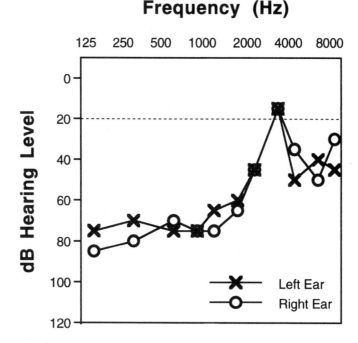

Figure 10–3. Pure-tone air-conduction thresholds for a patient with bilateral auditory neuropathy.

Speech recognition bilaterally was poor in quiet and in noise. Word recognition showed maximum discrimination scores of 14% and 20% for monosyllables in quiet for the right and left ears, respectively. These scores are poorer than would be expected if the loss were cochlear in nature (Yellin, Jerger, & Fifer, 1989). Masking level difference testing showed no release of masking when the phase of the noise was shifted. Test results are summarized in Table 10–1.

Auditory brain stem, middle latency responses, and late (N1-P2) cortical potentials all showed poor synchrony. Radiologic test results (CT and MRI) showed no lesions or abnormalities of the auditory nerve or brain stem.

This patient has consistently shown robust transient evoked (Figure 10–4) and distortion product OAEs which are inconsistent with the audiometric configuration. Efferent suppression of TEOAEs was absent for binaural, ipsilateral, and contralateral broadband noise suppressors. Figure 10–5 displays the EchoMaster summary of suppression for the binaural noise condition for this patient. What is readily apparent is the lack of suppression (straight lines at zero) for both amplitude and time.

Table 10–1. Summary of test results for a patient with bilateral auditory neuropathy.

Test	Results
Pure-tone thresholds	Moderately severe rising to normal to mild range, bilaterally symmetric
Speech recognition in quiet	Poor bilaterally
Speech recognition in noise	0% for words and sentences
Otoacoustic emissions	Normal bilaterally
Tympanograms	Normal bilaterally
Middle ear muscle reflexes	
Ipsilateral	Absent
Contralateral	Absent
Nonacoustic	Present
Cochlear microphonic	Present (inverts with stimulus polarity reversal)
Auditory brain stem response	Absent bilaterally
Middle latency response	Absent bilaterally
Late response (N1–P2)	Abnormal bilaterally
Masking level difference (MLD)	No MLD (i.e., 0 dB) bilaterally
Efferent suppression of TEOAEs	No suppression for binaural, ipsilateral, or contralateral suppressors for either ear

Furthermore, comparison of suppression amplitude between 8 and 18 ms for binaural, ipsilateral, and contralateral suppressors in this patient to normal individuals shows that this patient is well below the normal range, particularly for binaural noise (Figure 10–6).

An absent ABR in the presence of normal OAEs is a classic indicator of an auditory dys-synchrony/neuropathy. Absent middle ear muscle reflexes, ABRs and middle latency responses suggest abnormal neural synchrony or processing of information from the lower brain stem, thalamus, and primary auditory areas. The lack of efferent suppression of OAEs is consistent with abnormalities affecting the auditory nerve or caudal brain stem. Although this patient did not have synchronous cortical potentials, some auditory neuropathy patients do show quite normal cortical responses, consistent with successful cortical integration.

Case Study 2: Unilateral Auditory Dys-Synchrony/Neuropathy and Abnormal Efferent Suppression of TEOAEs

This patient was referred to us at age 12 years with reported learning problems thought to be related to a central auditory disorder. She had not

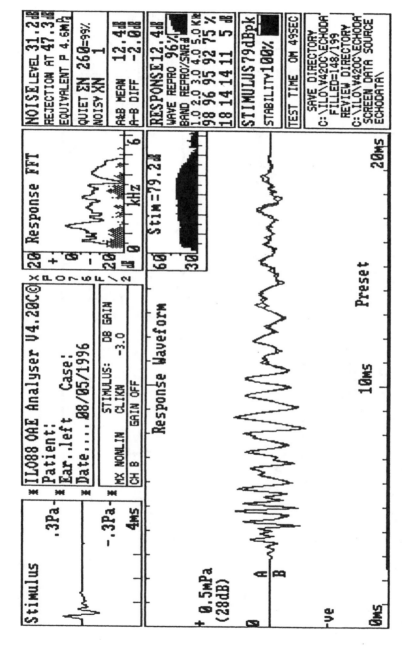

Figure 10–4. Transient-evoked otoacoustic emissions for a patient with bilateral auditory neuropathy. *(continued)*

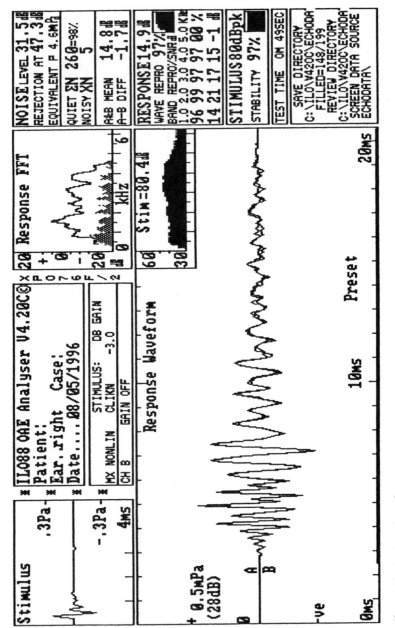

Figure 10–4. *(continued)*

194

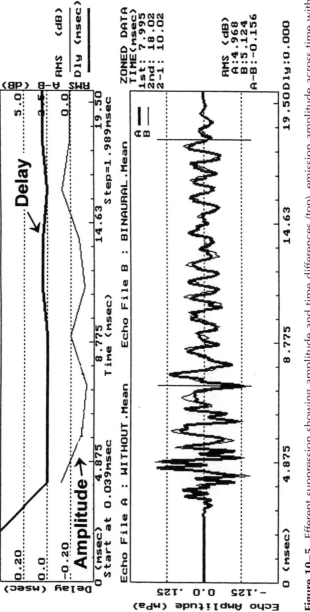

Figure 10–5. Efferent suppression showing amplitude and time differences (top), emission amplitude across time with and without suppressor noise (bottom) for a patient with bilateral auditory neuropathy. Emission amplitude in the bracketed region (8–18 ms, bottom) is 4.97 dB without noise and 5.12 with noise.

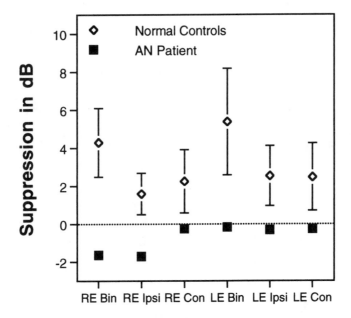

Test Condition

Figure 10–6. Comparison of suppression amplitude in the 8 to 18 ms time range for a patient with bilateral auditory neuropathy/dys-synchrony and a group of normal individuals. Effects of binaural, ipsilateral, and contralateral noise are shown.

complained of a hearing loss, and the abnormality was first noted on a hearing screening test at her school.

Audiometric testing indicated normal pure-tone thresholds across the frequency range for the right ear and a profound loss for the left ear, with no response to pure tones in that ear with appropriate masking in the normal ear (Figure 10–7). Word recognition in quiet was consistent with the hearing loss (i.e., 100% in the right ear and 0% in the left ear). Ipsilateral and contralateral middle ear muscle reflexes were normal upon stimulation of the right ear and absent for stimulation of the left ear. The auditory brain stem response was normal for the right ear and absent for the left ear. Test findings are summarized in Table 10–2.

To this point, all test results for this patient were consistent with a unilateral cochlear hearing loss of unknown origin. However, OAEs were present and robust for both ears, as were CM that inverted with reversal of the stimulus polarity. These findings were consistent with normal outer hair cell function bilaterally and the presence of auditory neuropathy/dys-synchrony in the left ear.

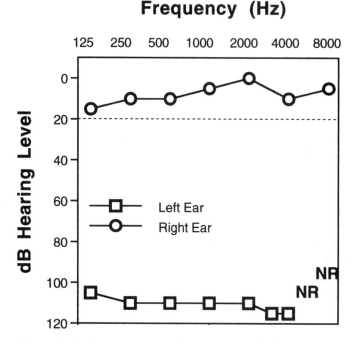

Figure 10–7. Pure-tone air-conduction thresholds for a patient with unilateral auditory neuropathy/dys-synchrony.

The efferent suppression patterns found for binaural, ipsilateral, and contralateral noise provide insight into the influence of afferent and efferent pathways on suppression in this patient. When the right (normal) ear received the suppressor stimulus (the RE Bin, RE Ipsi, and LE Con conditions shown in Figure 10–8), suppression was either within the normal range or, in the case of RE Ipsi, greater than normal. In contrast, when the left (profound loss ear) received the suppressor stimulus, suppression was below normal regardless of the click location

IS THIS AN AFFERENT LACK OF SYNCHRONY OR A LACK OF EFFERENT CONNECTIONS?

In patients with bilateral auditory neuropathy, the lack of suppression of TEOAEs makes it difficult to separate possible contributions of afferent and efferent pathways. Results from patients with unilateral neuropathy shed light on this question, however. Our observations on this unilateral auditory neuropathy patient indicate that the efferent system is functioning

Table 10–2. Summary of test results for a patient with unilateral auditory neuropathy.

Test	Results
Pure-tone thresholds	Right ear: normal Left ear: profound hearing loss
Speech recognition in quiet	Right ear: normal Left ear: 0% for words and sentences
Otoacoustic emissions	Normal bilaterally
Tympanograms	Normal bilaterally
Middle ear muscle reflexes Right ear stimulated Left ear stimulated	 Normal Absent
Cochlear microphonic (CM)	Present bilaterally
Auditory brain stem response	Right ear: normal Left ear: absent
Efferent suppression of transient evoked otoacoustic emissions (TEOAEs)	RE Stim—RE Rec: Present (large) RE Stim—LE Rec: Present (small) LE Stim—RE Rec: No suppression LE Stim—LE Rec: No suppression Both Stim—RE Rec: Present (large, = ipsi) Both Stim—LE Rec: Present (small)

Note. LE = left ear; RE = right ear; Rec = ear recording TEOAE; Stim = ear stimulated with suppressor.

even on the profound hearing loss ear side and can be partially activated by noise to the good (right) ear (see Table 10–2). When the poor (left) ear was stimulated, however, no efferent function in either the right or left ear was recordable. Similarly, noise delivered binaurally did suppress the emissions on the left side, although only about as much as simply monaural right ear noise.

SUMMARY

This chapter describes characteristics of efferent suppression of otoacoustic emissions in normal individuals and in patients with auditory dyssynchrony/neuropathy. Efferent suppression of TEOAEs is observed in all individuals with normal auditory function when appropriate recording and analysis methods are used. Efferent suppression is not typically

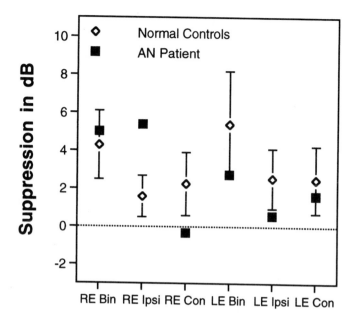

Figure 10–8. Comparison of suppression amplitude in the 8 to 18 ms time range for a patient with unilateral auditory neuropathy and a group of normal individuals. Effects of binaural, ipsilateral, and contralateral noise are shown.

present and appears to be a sensitive measure of auditory function in patients with auditory dys-synchrony/neuropathy and should provide insight into the underlying mechanisms.

Acknowledgments: Research at Kresge Hearing Research Laboratory is supported by the NIH National Institute on Deafness and Other Communication Disorders, U.S. Department of Defense, American Hearing Research Foundation, National Organization for Hearing Research, Deafness Research Foundation, Oberkotter Foundation, Kam's Fund for Hearing Research, Marriott Foundation, and the Louisiana Lions Eye Foundation. Contributions to the studies at Kresge Hearing Research Laboratory on efferent suppression and auditory neuropathy were made by the following individuals: Harriet Berlin, M.A., Jill Bordelon, M.C.D., Shanda Brashears, M.C.D., Leah Goforth-Barter, M.S., Annette Hurley, M.S., Jennifer Jean-freau, M.C.D., Elizabeth Montgomery, M.S., Thierry Morlet, Ph.D., Patti St. John, M.A., Sonya Tedesco, M.C.D., Han Wen, M.S.B.E., and Diane Wilensky, M.A.

APPENDIX

Some Web sites with information related to auditory neuropathy and patient management:

Information on the evaluation and management of auditory dyssynchrony/neuropathy from Kresge Hearing Research Laboratory, Department of Otolaryngology, LSU Health Sciences Center: http://www.kresgelab.org under the section titled "Information About Deafness."

The EchoMaster efferent suppression analysis program can be downloaded from the Kresge lab Web site: http://www.kresgelab.org.

REFERENCES

Berlin, C. I., Bordelon, J., St. John, P., Wilensky, D., Hurley, A., Kluka, E., & Hood, L. J. (1998). Reversing click polarity may uncover auditory neuropathy in infants. *Ear and Hearing, 19*, 37–47.

Berlin, C. I., Hood, L. J., Cecola, R. P., Jackson, D. F., & Szabo P. (1993). Does Type I afferent neuron dysfunction reveal itself through lack of efferent suppression? *Hearing Research, 65*, 40–50.

Berlin, C. I., Hood, L. J., Hurley, A., & Wen, H. (1994). Contralateral suppression of otoacoustic emissions: An index of the function of the medial olivocochlear system. *Otolaryngology—Head and Neck Surgery, 100*, 3–21.

Berlin, C. I., Hood, L. J., Hurley, A., Wen, H., & Kemp, D. T. (1995). Bilateral noise suppresses click-evoked otoacoustic emissions more than ipsilateral or contralateral noise. *Hearing Research, 87*, 96–103.

Berlin, C. I., Hood, L. J., Wen, H., Szabo, P., Cecola, R. P., Rigby, P., & Jackson, D. F. (1993). Contralateral suppression of non-linear click-evoked otoacoustic emissions. *Hearing Research, 71*, 1–11.

Berlin, C. I., Szabo, P., Cecola, P., Hood, L. J., Rigby, P., Erato, R., Fontenot, C., & Allen, J. (1991). Comparison of evoked otoacoustic emissions and distortion product emissions via the Kemp and cubic distortion product systems. *ARO Abstracts, 14*, 66.

Brown, M. C., & Nuttall, A. L. (1984). Efferent control of cochlear inner hair cell response in the guinea pig. *Journal of Physiology, 354*, 625–646.

Buno, W., Jr. (1978). Auditory nerve fiber activity influenced by contralateral sound stimulation. *Experimental Neurology, 59*, 62–74.

Collet, L., Kemp, D. T., Veuillet, E., Duclaux, R., Moulin, A., & Morgon, A. (1990). Effect of contralateral auditory stimuli on active cochlear micro-mechanical properties in human subjects. *Hearing Research, 43*, 251–262.

Folsom, R. C., & Owsley, R. M. (1987). N1 action potentials in humans. *Acta Otolaryngologica (Stockholm), 103*, 262–265.

Galambos, R. (1956). Suppression of auditory nerve activity by stimulation of efferent fibers to the cochlea. *Journal of Neurophysiology, 19*, 424–437.

Giraud, A. L., Collet, L., Chery-Croze, S., Magnan, J., & Chays, A. (1995). Evidence of a medial olivocochlear involvement in contralateral suppression of otoacoustic emissions in humans. *Brain Research, 705,* 15–23.

Gorga, M. P., Stelmachowicz, P. G., Barlow, S. M., & Brookhouser, P. E. (1995). Case of recurrent, reversible, sudden sensorineural hearing loss in a child. *Journal of the American Academy of Audiology, 6,* 163–172.

Grose, J. H. (1983). The effect of contralateral suppression on spontaneous acoustic emissions. *Journal of the Acoustical Society of America, 74,* S38.

Hood, L. J., Berlin, C. I., Bordelon, J., Goforth-Barter, L., Hurley, A., & Tedesco, S. (2000). Patients with auditory neuropathy lack efferent suppression of transient evoked otoacoustic emissions. *ARO Abstracts, 23,* 159.

Hood, L. J., Berlin, C. I., Hurley, A., Cecola, R. P., & Bell, B. (1996). Contralateral suppression of click-evoked otoacoustic emissions: Intensity effects. *Hearing Research, 101,* 113–118.

Kaga, K., Nakamura, M., Shinogami, M., Tsuzuku, T., Yamada, K., & Shindo, M. (1996). Auditory nerve disease of both ears revealed by auditory brainstem responses, electrocochleography and otoacoustic emissions. *Scandinavian Audiology, 25,* 233–238.

Kawase, T., & Takasaka, T. (1995). The effects contralateral noise on masked compound action potentials in humans. *Hearing Research, 91,* 1–6.

Kemp, D. T. (1978). Stimulated acoustic emissions from within the human auditory system. *Journal of the Acoustical Society of America, 64,* 1386–1391.

Kemp, D. T., & Chum, R. (1980). Properties of the generator of stimulated acoustic emissions. *Hearing Research, 2,* 213–232.

Liang, F., Liu, C., & Liu, B. (1997). Otoacoustic emission and auditory efferent function testing in patients with sensori-neural hearing loss. *Chinese Medical Journal, 110,* 139–41.

Liberman, M. C. (1989). Rapid assessment of sound-evoked olivocochlear feedback: Suppression of compound action potentials by contralateral sound. *Hearing Research, 38,* 47–56.

Maison, S., Micheyl, C., & Collet, L. (1998). Contralateral frequency-modulated tones suppress transient-evoked otoacoustic emissions in humans. *Hearing Research, 117,* 114–118.

Maurer, J., Beck, W., Mann, W., & Mintert, R. (1992). Veränderungen otoakustischer Emissionen unto gleichzeitiger Beschallung des Gegenohres bei Normalpersonen und bei Patientien mit einseitigem Akustikusneurinom. [Changes of amplitude of otoacoustic emissions under contralateral noise in normal hearing persons and in patients with unilateral acoustic neuroma.] *Laryngology-Rhinology-Otology, 71,* 69–73.

Mott, J. B., Norton, S. J., Neely, S. T., & Warr, W. B. (1989). Changes in spontaneous otoacoustic emissions produced by acoustic stimulation of the contralateral ear. *Hearing Research, 38,* 229–242.

Moulin, A., Collet, L., & Duclaux, R. (1993). Contralateral auditory stimulation alters acoustic distortion products in humans. *Hearing Research, 65,* 193–210.

Moulin, A., Collet, L., & Morgon, A. (1992). Influence of spontaneous otoacoustic emissions (SOAE) on acoustic distortion product input/output functions: Does the medial efferent system act differently in the vicinity of an SOAE? *Acta Oto-Laryngologica, 112,* 210–214.

Mountain, D. C. (1980). Changes in endolymphatic potential and crossed olivo-cochlear bundle stimulation alter cochlear mechanics. *Science, 210,* 71–72.

Nieschall, M., Beneking, R., & Stoll, W. (1997). Increased amplitude of distortion product emissions in the human caused by contralateral low intensity acoustic stimulation. *HNO, 45,* 378–384.

Prasher, D., Ryan, S., & Luxon, L. (1994). Contralateral suppression of transiently evoked otoacoustic emission and neuro-otology. *British Journal of Audiology, 28,* 247–254.

Puel, J.-L., & Rebillard, G. (1990). Effect of contralateral sound stimulation on the distortion product 2F1-F2: Evidence that the medial efferent system is involved. *Journal of the Acoustical Society of America, 87,* 1630–1635.

Rabinowitz, W. M., & Widen, G. P. (1984). Interaction of spontaneous otoacoustic emissions and external sounds. *Journal of the Acoustical Society of America, 76,* 1713–1720.

Ryan, S., & Kemp, D. T. (1996). The influence of evoking stimulus level on the neural suppression of transient evoked otoacoustic emissions. *Hearing Research, 94,* 140–147.

Ryan, S., Kemp, D. T., & Hinchcliffe, R. (1991). The influence of contralateral acoustic stimulation on click-evoked otoacoustic emissions in humans. *British Journal of Audiology, 25,* 391–397.

Schloth, E., & Zwicker, E. (1983). Mechanical and acoustic influences on spontaneous otoacoustic emission. *Hearing Research, 11,* 285–293.

Starr, A., McPherson, D., Patterson, J., Don, M., Luxford, W., Shannon, R., Sininger, Y. S., Tonokawa, L., & Waring, M. (1991). Absence of both auditory evoked potentials and auditory percepts depending on timing cues. *Brain, 114,* 1157–1180.

Starr, A., Picton, T. W., Sininger, Y. S., Hood, L. J., & Berlin, C. I. (1996). Auditory neuropathy. *Brain, 119,* 741–753.

Timpe-Syverson, G. K., & Decker, T. N. (1999). Attention effects on distortion-product otoacoustic emissions with contralateral speech stimuli. *Journal of the American Academy of Audiology, 10,* 371–378.

Veuillet, E., Collet, L., & Duclaux, R. (1991). Effect of contralateral acoustic stimulation on active cochlear micromechanical properties in human subjects: Dependence on stimulus variables. *Journal of Neurophysiology, 65,* 724–735.

Warr, W. B., & Guinan, J. J. (1978). Efferent innervation of the organ of Corti: Two different systems. *Brain Research, 173,* 152–155.

Warr, W. B., Guinan, J. J., & White, J. S. (1986). Organization of the efferent fibers: The lateral and medial olivocochlear systems. In R. A. Altschuler, R. P. Bobbin, & D. W. Hoffman (Eds.), *Neurobiology of hearing: The cochlea.* New York: Raven Press.

Wen, H., Berlin, C. I., Hood, L. J., Jackson, D., & Hurley, A. (1993). A program for the quantification and analysis of transient evoked otoacoustic emissions. *ARO Abstracts, 16,* 102.

Williams, E. A., Brookes, G. B., & Prasher, D. K. (1993). Effects of contralateral acoustic stimulation on otoacoustic emissions following vestibular neurectomy. *Scandinavian Audiology, 22,* 197–203.

Williams, E. A., Brookes, G. B., & Prasher, D. K. (1994). Effects of olivocochlear bundle section on otoacoustic emissions in humans: Efferent effects in comparison with control subjects. *Acta Otolaryngologica, 114,* 121–129.

Yellin, M. W., Jerger, J., & Fifer, R. C. (1989). Norms for disproportionate loss in speech intelligibility. *Ear and Hearing, 10,* 231–234.

Cochlear Implantation of Patients With Auditory Neuropathy

Patricia Trautwein, Jon Shallop, Lee Fabry, and Rick Friedman

Management of patients with auditory neuropathy (AN) is challenging for clinicians and physicians alike because of the heterogeneity of the populations' audiologic and neurologic findings, in addition to the uncertain etiology and pathophysiology. Audiometric testing reveals hearing loss of varying degrees from mild to profound. One pervasive observation with AN is degraded speech perception, ranging from limited to no open-set discrimination regardless of the degree of hearing loss. Trials with conventional forms of amplification (hearing aids, FM systems, or tactile aids) have demonstrated limited success (see Cone-Wesson, Rance, & Sininger, Chapter 12, this volume). Furthermore, the effectiveness of amplification may not be directly related to audiometric thresholds (i.e., a patient with audiometric thresholds in the severe range may demonstrate more benefit with amplification than a patient with thresholds in the mild range; Rance et al., 1999).

For children with AN, development of auditory and oral communication skills are compromised. Nonetheless, because comprehension typically improves dramatically in the auditory plus visual modality, these children routinely are referred to educational programs with an emphasis on manual (visual) modes of communication. Approximately one third of the patients with AN have audiometric thresholds in the severe-to-profound range (Sininger, Trautwein, Shallop, Fabry, & Starr, 1999). Children with hearing loss in the severe-to-profound range that results from a variety of etiologies and who do not receive benefit from amplification are considered cochlear implant candidates. This chapter will address the possible benefits and drawbacks of cochlear implantation for children with AN.

Cochlear implantation is routinely performed in patients with sensory losses in which the cochlea is the primary site of dysfunction, although the status of the auditory nerve remains elusive. In cases of AN, a variety of potential sites of dysfunction has been proposed. Harrison (1998, and Chapter 4 in this volume) has suggested a cochlear origin for AN in which the inner hair cells or the synaptic connection to the inner hair cells are the source of dysfunction. If the site of dysfunction is cochlear, an implant may be a viable compensation as it is in cases of sensory hearing loss. Others have postulated that the site of dysfunction is not cochlear in origin, but lies at the level of the auditory nerve. In Chapter 3 of this volume, Starr provides evidence that AN can be caused by auditory nerve (axonal) degeneration or demyelination. The resulting lack of neural synchrony and poor temporal encoding accounts for the grossly abnormal or absent auditory brain stem response (ABR) and degraded speech perception (Zeng, Oba, Garde, Sininger, & Starr, 1999). Because of the suggested pathology of the auditory nerve, the efficacy of cochlear implantation could be questioned for these patients; however, research has, in fact, supported the use of electrical stimulation in cases of auditory nerve dysfunction. Zhou, Abbas, and Assouline (1995) reported that electrical stimulation produces synchronous ABRs in the presence of peripheral auditory nerve demyelination. This suggests that the electrical stimulation of a cochlear implant could provide reliable, consistent neural firing even in the presence of a diseased peripheral nerve. If electrical stimulation can normalize the timing of firing patterns in the auditory nerve and at higher levels, the result should be better speech perception (see Zeng et al., Chapter 8 this volume). In addition, electrical stimulation provided by the cochlear implant may even promote neural survival (Araki et al., 1998; Mitchell et al., 1997) and restore temporal encoding (Shannon, 1993).

Although the potential benefits of cochlear implantation are promising, drawbacks do exist. The standard risks of the surgical procedure and anesthesia remain but are no greater for children with AN than for children with sensory hearing loss. Research has suggested that the insertion of the electrode array may damage cochlear structures and destroy residual hearing (Gstoettner et al., 1997; O'Leary, Fayed, House, & Linthicum, 1991). If that is the case, then the implantation procedure may damage structures in the cochlea (i.e., the outer hair cells), which seem to be functioning normally in many patients with AN. Of course, in all cases, implantation is no guarantee for the development of oral speech communication skills. All families need to be counseled appropriately to assure reasonable expectations regarding the outcome of any cochlear implant.

Certainly, before the accurate diagnosis of AN was uncovered, patients with the disorder received cochlear implants based on severe-to-profound audiometric thresholds and unsuccessful trials with conventional amplification. Occasionally, it is possible to identify these patients after the fact and assess cochlear implant benefit. One such case is illustrated below in addition to six cases in which the diagnosis of AN was made before implantation. These case studies serve as a limited example of the range of potential benefit children with AN may experience with a cochlear implant.

CHILD A

This is a summary of a case presented by Trautwein, Sininger, and Nelson (2000). This male child was the product of a healthy, full-term pregnancy. Physical developmental milestones were reached at age-appropriate times. When the development of speech and language appeared delayed, however, the family suspected a hearing loss. Child A was 18 months of age when diagnosed with a severe-to-profound hearing loss following a no-response ABR. He was immediately fit with high-gain, conventional amplification and enrolled in an oral preschool for children with hearing loss. Despite the consistent use of amplification and intensive auditory training, auditory-oral language skills did not improve. Therefore, the family was referred for a cochlear implant evaluation.

At the time of the cochlear implant preevaluation, the child was 2 years, 11 months old. As seen in Figure 11–1, unaided, behavioral audiometric thresholds were obtained in the severe-to-profound range. For both ears, aided thresholds were within the long-term average speech spectrum (LTASS; Ling, 1978) through 1000 Hz in both ears. Immittance measures revealed normal tympanograms and absent acoustic reflexes. These results were consistent with previous assessments. Although functional gain measures demonstrated substantial improvement in aided over unaided conditions, speech perception testing revealed no open- or closed-set speech discrimination in the binaurally aided condition.

Transient evoked otoacoustic emissions (TEOAEs) were obtained for the first time during the cochlear implant preevaluation. TEOAEs were clearly absent for the left ear (Figure 11–2A) but appeared to be present in the right ear (Figure 11–2B) and warranted further testing. A repeat ABR in response to condensation and rarefaction clicks revealed an absent neural response with a present cochlear microphonic (CM) for both ears (depicted in Figure 11–3). The CM appears more robust in the right ear, which also showed an emission. The use of amplification was temporarily discontinued in the right ear, and robust TEOAEs were subsequently recorded as shown in Figure 11–2C. Data from our facility suggest that the incidence of unilateral AN is rare (see Chapter 2 by Sininger and Oba in

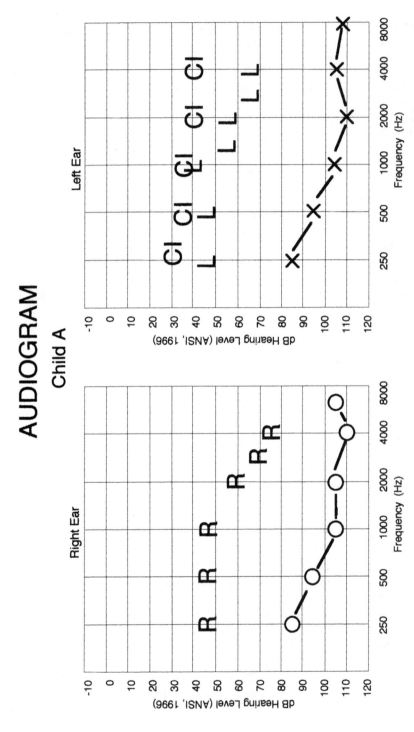

Figure 11–1. Unaided (O and X) and aided (right, left, and cochlear implant [R, L, CI]) for Child A pre- and postimplantation.

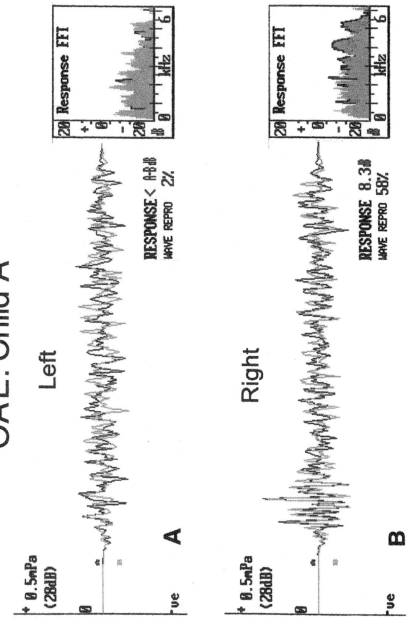

Figure 11–2. Initial recording of the transient evoked otoacoustic emissions (A and B) and repeat recording for the right ear (C) for Child A.

(continued)

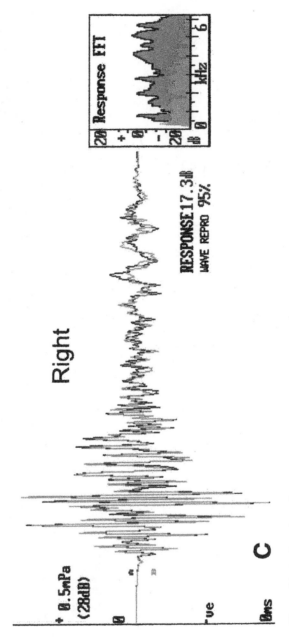

Figure 11–2. *(continued)*

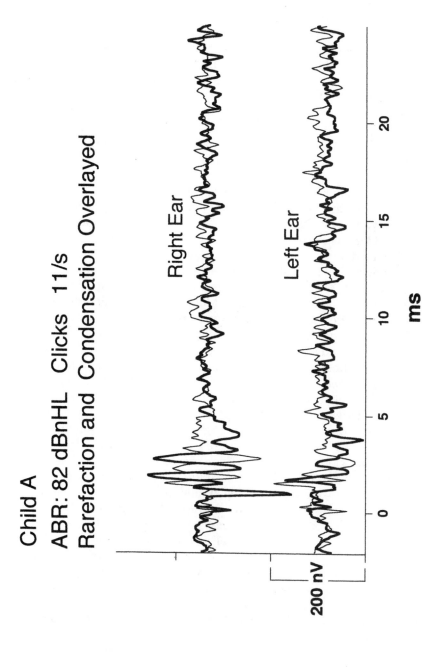

Figure 11–3. Auditory brain stem response recording with condensation and rarefaction click stimuli for Child A.

this volume). Therefore, the presence of CM and OAE in one ear was taken as sufficient evidence to support a diagnosis of bilateral AN.

The cochlear implant team and the parents, with guarded expectations, decided to proceed with the implantation of Cochlear Corporation's Nucleus CI24M device. The left ear was selected for implantation because of its lack of measurable emissions. The child was 3 years, 3 months of age at the time of implantation. Surgery was uncomplicated, and a full electrode insertion was achieved. Following a brief recovery period, the child was fit with the externally worn speech processor programmed according the SPEAK speech processing strategy (McKay, McDermott, Vandali, & Clark, 1992; Skinner, Clark, Whitford, Seligman, & Staller, 1994). Audiometric thresholds with the cochlear implant, as seen in Figure 11–1, were within the LTASS.

Child A remained in an oral education program and received intensive auditory training. Following 1 year of implant use, his speech perception skills were reevaluated. Recall that before implantation, it was determined that this child had no closed- or open-set speech discrimination. In fact, he did not even demonstrate pattern perception or phoneme discrimination without visual cues. At the 1 year postevaluation, the Early Speech Perception Test (ESP) and the Test of Auditory Comprehension (TAC) were administered. The ESP test (Moog & Geers, 1990) is designed to be used with children having limited vocabulary and language skills to assess speech perception ability. The test consists of three sets of test stimuli, each administered as a closed set. Test results allow for the placement of children into four speech perception categories: 1 = *no pattern perception,* 2 = *pattern perception,* 3 = *some word identification,* and 4 = *consistent word identification.* After 1 year of cochlear implant use, Child A is in category 4: consistent word identification. This suggests that the cochlear implant has permitted some degree of speech perception. The TAC (Trammell & Owens, 1977) is a comprehensive auditory discrimination test administered in a taped, closed-set format. There are 10 subtests arranged in a hierarchical order evaluating a range of abilities including suprasegmental discrimination, memory-sequencing abilities for up to four critical elements, auditory comprehension, and auditory figure-ground abilities. Before implantation, this child could not pass the first subtest without visual cues. After only 1 year of cochlear implant use, this child with AN passed the third subtest, which indicates a child's ability to discriminate stereotypic messages. Child A's overall progress with the implant falls within the wide range of performance seen in all other children with cochlear implants (Cohen, Waltzman, Roland, Staller, & Hoffman, 1999; Miyamoto, Kirk, Svirsky, & Sehgal, 1999; O'Donoghue, Nikolopoulos, Archbold, & Tait, 1998). Subjectively, his therapists report improvement in daily listening skills and an expansion in both receptive and expressive vocabulary. The parents are very pleased with his progress.

CHILD B

This female child was the first known case of binaural auditory neuropathy at Mayo Clinic in Rochester, Minnesota. She had a normal prenatal history including labor, delivery, early growth, and motor development. There was no history of otitis media or ototoxic drugs. In June 1995, when Child B was 15 months old, her parents brought her to the Otorhinolaryngology Department at Mayo Clinic for a hearing evaluation, because of delayed speech and language development. The results of her general pediatric, ophthalmologic, otorhinolaryngologic, and pediatric neurologic exams were all within normal limits. All the screening laboratory studies including complete blood count, electrolyte, serum thyroxin, and syphilis serology were negative or normal. A magnetic resonance imaging study with contrast was performed with sedation and interpreted to be within the normal range.

The behavioral audiogram shown in Figure 11–4 for Child B revealed a profound bilateral hearing loss. Tympanograms revealed normal middle ear pressure and compliance, and acoustic reflexes were absent in both ears. Transient evoked otoacoustic emissions were present bilaterally as seen in Figure 11–5. An AR revealed no synchronous neural activity; however, a CM was apparent as seen in Figure 11–6. This child was therefore diagnosed with auditory neuropathy.

Child B was provided with a tactile aid and responded reasonably well to tactile stimulation. The team at Mayo Clinic initially elected not to recommend a cochlear implant because of the lack of reports in the literature of successful implantation of patients with AN. The parents were counseled to adopt cued speech as the preferred communication mode for their child (see Cone-Wesson et al. Chapter 12 in this volume for an explanation of cued speech). The family received private tutoring in cued speech and rapidly acquired fluency with this methodology.

Child B was enrolled in an oral preschool program and underwent a trial with powerful hearing aids with careful audiologic monitoring and measurements of otoacoustic emissions. She realized little gain and received only minimal benefit from the hearing aids as shown in Figure 11–4 and it was noted that her emissions would temporarily diminish or disappear whenever she used the hearing aid. At the end of the school year, the parents again considered the possibility of a cochlear implant. Case B's speech and language skills had progressed dramatically, but she clearly needed additional auditory input beyond her hearing aids to succeed in oral education. She returned to the Mayo Clinic for a cochlear implant evaluation. She continued to demonstrate the presence of bilateral OAEs and absent ABR. Computerized tomography scan demonstrated patent cochleae with normal internal auditory canals. The team and parents decided to proceed with the implantation of the Cochlear Corporation's

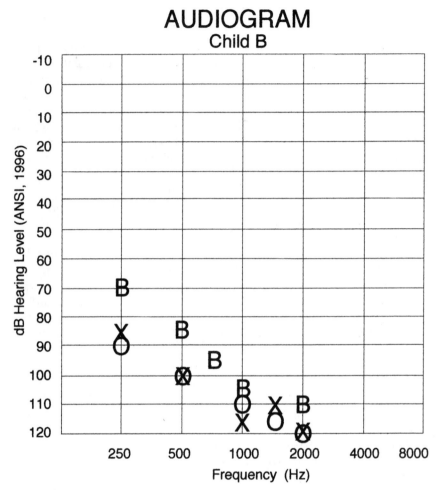

Figure 11–4. Unaided (O for right ear and X for left ear) and binaurally aided (B) audiometric findings for child B before implantation.

Nucleus CI24M device in the right ear. At that time the child was 4 years, 5 months old.

At the initial fitting of the speech processor, a program map utilizing the SPEAK strategy was created and activated. She was quiet and somewhat apprehensive when first listening to sound. After several minutes, she became comfortable with her cochlear implant, and informal testing could be conducted using items from the ESP test including a ball and a plastic ice-cream cone. These words and objects were presented using both

OAE: Child B

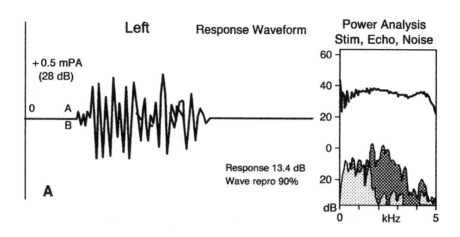

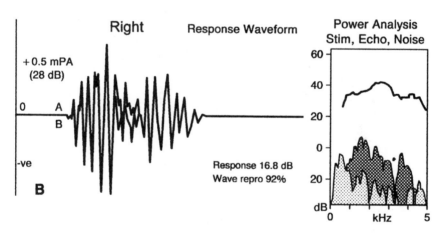

Figure 11–5. Transient evoked otoacoustic emission recordings for Child B.

vision and hearing. After she could point to the object requested using auditory and visual presentation, the task was repeated using audition alone. She was able to perform this task correctly three times out of five, which indicated auditory awareness of speech pattern contrasts by the end of the first day. On the second and third programming days, maps were refined further and levels were adjusted to avoid any adverse reactions.

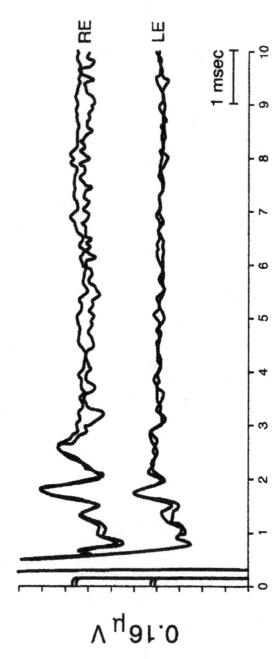

Figure 11–6. Auditory brain stem response recording for Child B.

Child B continued in an oral education program for the first year of implant use. She has made remarkable progress in her speech and language development to the point that during her first annual evaluation, she scored 64% words and 75% phonemes correct on the Kindergarten Phonetically Balanced Word Test (PBK; Haskins, 1949). Although her parents occasionally supplement communication with cued speech, she is considered an "oral" child who responds readily to auditory-only presentations from her parents, teachers, and others. Child B is now "mainstreamed" in public school kindergarten for the morning, and in the afternoon, she attends the oral program for additional oral education and auditory skills training. It is remarkable this child has made such good progress enabling this educational plan only 12 months after receiving a cochlear implant. Her preimplant oral training and especially the intensive use of cued speech have enabled her to reach high levels of oral language skills.

CHILD C

This child is the younger male sibling of Child B. He was brought to Mayo Clinic for evaluation when he was 5 months of age after his sister was diagnosed with AN. Prenatal history, labor, and delivery were normal. Results of his general pediatric, otorhinolaryngology, ophthalmologic, and pediatric neurologic evaluations were also normal. A magnetic resonance imaging study with contrast was negative.

The audiogram for Child C (shown in Figure 11–7) revealed a profound, bilateral hearing loss. There was no synchronous neural activity in the ABR for either ear; however, a prominent CM is seen in the recording as shown in Figure 11–8. Otoacoustic emissions were present bilaterally and quite large as seen in Figure 11–9. Amplification trials with a tactile aid and conventional hearing aids were unsuccessful. The communication mode selected by the parents of Child C was oral, utilizing cued speech. He was enrolled in an oral education program. After the successful cochlear implantation of his older sibling, Child C was evaluated for a cochlear implant. Implantation of the right ear with a Nucleus CI24M was performed when the child was 3 years, 6 months of age. At initial programming, maps were created utilizing the SPEAK processing strategy.

Child C continued in an oral education program following implantation. He is in a class of four other children with cochlear implants. At home, the parents use cued speech. Child C is making slower progress in speech and language development compared with his older sister. He has definite sound detection skills, and he is able to perform closed-set auditory-only word identification tasks from sets of six objects with an accuracy of 80%.

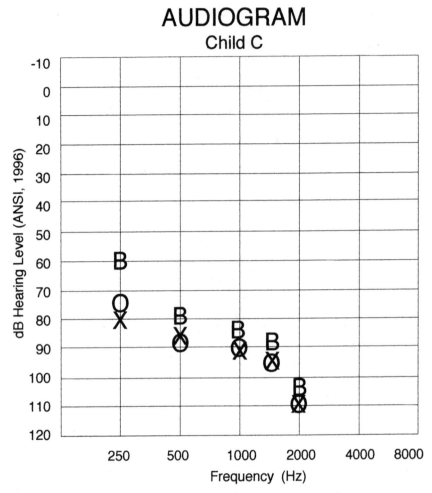

Figure 11–7. Unaided (O for right ear and X for left ear) and binaurally aided (B) audiometric findings for child C before implantation.

CHILD D

This child was initially seen at Mayo Clinic at the age of 4 years 2 months. He had been referred for evaluation and the possibility of a cochlear implant. He was extensively evaluated before being referred to Mayo and is described as subject GP in Stein et al. (1996). Child D's prenatal history was apparently normal, but his parents were Rh incompatible. He was also the product of a premature delivery. At birth, he was noted to have hyperbilirubinemia requiring exchange transfusion.

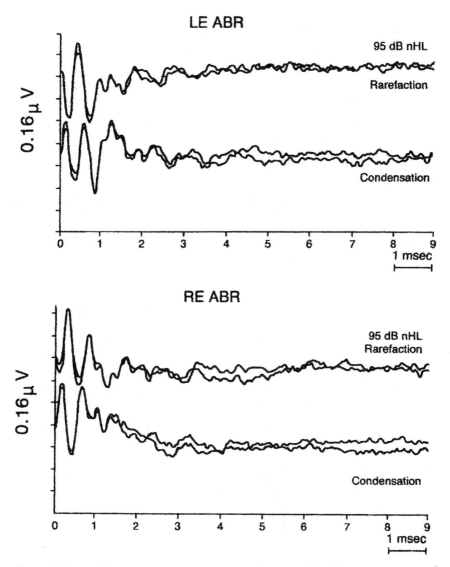

Figure 11–8. Auditory brain stem response recordings for Child C.

Child D was noted to have a hearing loss at the age of 5 months when an abnormal ABR was seen. At the same time, he "passed" an otoacoustic emissions screening test. In addition, he had frequent bouts of otitis media that were treated with myringotomy and ventilation tube insertion on three occasions. At the time of his initial diagnosis in Chicago, his parents followed recommendations to utilize cued speech. They also were

OAE: Child C

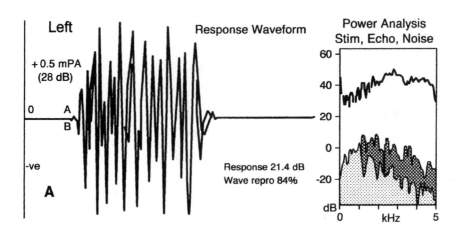

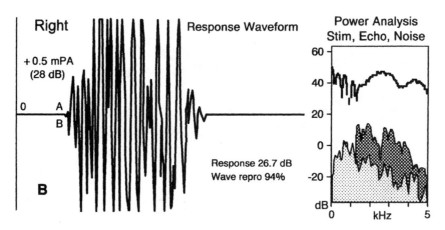

Figure 11–9. Transient evoked otoacoustic emission recordings for Child C.

encouraged to consider a cochlear implant because he had responded poorly to the use of powerful, behind-the-ear hearing aids.

When evaluated at the Mayo Clinic, Child D's tympanic membranes were noted to be retracted, and middle ear effusion was present. As shown in Figure 11–10, his audiogram demonstrated a severe-to-profound bilateral sensorineural hearing loss. The presence of the middle ear effusion precluded the conclusive measurement of transient and distortion prod-

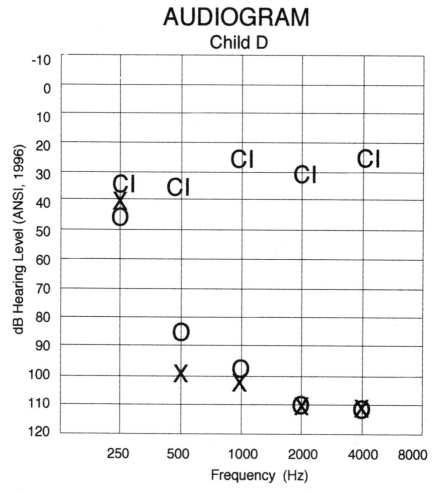

Figure 11–10. Unaided audiologic thresholds (O for right ear and X for left ear) before implantation and aided thresholds (CI) postimplantation for Child D.

uct otoacoustic emissions at that time. Imaging studies including magnetic resonance revealed no significant abnormality, and a computerized tomography scan demonstrated a patent cochlea bilaterally. After extensive consultations, a Cochlear Corporation Nucleus CI24m was implanted in the right ear. At the time of the surgery, just before the implantation, intra-operative electrocochleography recordings demonstrated absent neural responses with present CM, confirming the diagnosis of AN.

Initial stimulation and programming for Child D was approximately 3 weeks after surgery. Comfort and threshold levels were set utilizing behavioral responses to create a SPEAK map. Child D responded imme-diately to the sound and showed no adverse reactions. By the end of his first programming session, he was wearing the processor comfortably.

Child D is enrolled in an oral education program. He has made re-markable progress with his cochlear implant during his first year of hearing with the device. During an annual evaluation, he had a speech reception threshold using pictures of 35 dB HL with pure-tone aided thresholds within the LTASS as shown on Figure 11–10. On the early speech peception test, his scores placed him in category 4, indicating that he could demon-strate closed-set word recognition. His parents continue to report progress with open-set sentence recognition in daily living situations at home.

CHILD E

This female child received her Cochlear Corporation Nucleus 22 cochlear implant in 1995 at 3 years, 3 months of age following unsuccessful trial with power bilateral amplification. She was diagnosed with a severe hear-ing loss in the right ear and a profound hearing loss in the left ear as seen in Figure 11–11. Otoacoustic emissions testing was not performed at the time of her diagnosis, and initially the loss was thought to be cochlear in origin. She made significant progress in speech and language develop-ment following the first 2 years of cochlear implant use. It was not until her brother was born in 1996 that AN was suspected. Her brother's ABR evaluation revealed no neural response. Otoacoustic emissions were pres-ent for both ears, however, consistent with AN. Following her brother's diagnosis, recordings of OAEs were then obtained in child E's right ear, the nonimplant ear. Emissions were present, and a diagnosis of AN was made almost 3 years after she received the cochlear implant.

Child E's parents, teachers, and therapists report significant progress with the cochlear implant. Audiometric thresholds obtained with the im-plant are shown in Figure 11–11. At her 4-year postimplantation evalua-tion, she scored 56% correct on PBK words and passed subtest 5 (recalls two critical elements) on the TAC. She is mainstreamed for the first grade and receives support services as needed. Because she has made such significant progress, her younger brother was also implanted at 1 year, 9 months of age. Although he has only had the device a short time, he is reported to be doing well on informal testing.

CHILD F

Child F illustrates a child with auditory neuropathy in whom no speech perception benefit was obtained from cochlear implantation. This child

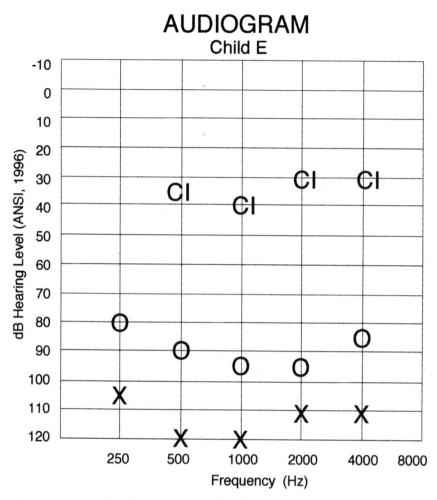

Figure 11–11. Unaided audiologic thresholds (O for right ear and X for left ear) before implantation and aided thresholds (CI) postimplantation for Child E.

was evaluated and followed by two major pediatric cochlear implant centers outside of the United States. Speech and language habilitation and educational management also took place outside of the United States. This boy, now 8 years old, was born at 33 weeks gestational age, at a birthweight of 2 kg and spent 5 weeks in neonatal intensive care. Medical records are not available from the neonatal period. Subsequent medical histories indicate that the neonatal course was otherwise unremarkable except that he was treated for hyperbilirubinemia with phototherapy.

The parents suspected hearing loss at 8 to 9 months of age. ABR tests completed at 11 months indicate no response, and further behavioral audiometric tests indicated a profound, bilateral hearing loss. Amplification with high-power behind-the-ear hearing aids was provided at 14 months, along with intensive auditory-verbal training and speech therapy. Child F commenced a preschool program that included children with normal hearing as well as children with other disabilities.

When Child F was nearly 2 years old, he had an electrocochleography evaluation performed with a transtympanic electrode under general anesthesia. In response to click stimulation of the left ear at 110 dB HL, there was no action potential; however a "large" positive summating potential (SP; O'Leary, Mitchell, Gibson, & Sanli, in press) was noted. This was also seen in response to tone pips as well as large cochlear microphonics. For the right ear, there was a "massive" positive SP for click stimulus levels of 70 dB HL and above but no AP at 110 dB HL. Also for the right ear, cochlear microphonics were present in response to tone-pip stimuli at octave intervals from 0.25–8 kHz at levels of 90 dB HL and above. Action potentials were reported present but only at 500 Hz and at 1 kHz at 100–110 dB HL. These results were interpreted by the otologist who performed the evaluation as "suggestive of a mixed cochlear and retrocochlear problem such as seen in kernicterus." Because of the abnormalities in the electrocochleography, implantation was not recommended at that time. Computerized tomography scans of the otic capsules completed at that time showed a normal left middle ear cleft, ossicular chain and bony cochlea, but some increased density of the external auditory canal and reduced aeration of the middle ear cleft for the right ear. The ossicular chain and cochlea had normal definition.

A newer model of powerful aids was fit at age 33 months. The audiogram obtained at age 3.5 years is shown in Figure 11–12, along with the aided results. Tympanometry results were within normal limits, but acoustic reflexes were absent

At 3.5 years of age, Child F was reevaluated for consideration of cochlear implantation. Speech perception and speech and language assessments were carried out. The results indicated limited use of auditory information, especially considering the use of amplification and the intensive speech and language therapy over a 2.5-year period. This child's left ear was implanted with the Cochlear Ltd CI–22 device just before his fourth birthday. The surgeon reported full insertion of the 22-channel electrode array. Electrically evoked ABRs were tested several weeks after implantation. They were reported as "an abnormal waveform with poor waves 2–5 and delays" and interpreted as evidence of lack of myelin and consistent with the preoperative electrocochleographic abnormalities.

Initial mapping sessions were reported to be noneventful, with the implant set in the BP+1 mode with 12 active electrodes (#19–4). Child F

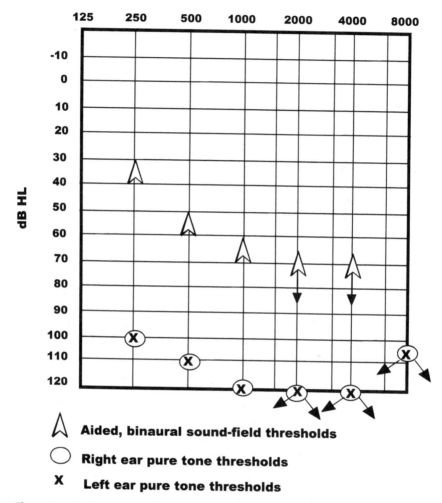

Figure 11–12. Pure tone audiogram and aided thresholds obtained when Child F was 3.5 years of age. There is no aided benefit for 2000–4000 Hz, although thresholds for low and midfrequencies show 50–55 dB of gain.

did not appear to be responsive to the stimuli provided by the implant, and within a few months, his map was changed to increase the area of stimulation across the array for each channel, first to BP+3 and later to BP+4.mode. After 2 months of experience with the BP+4 map, low-frequency vowel detection was reported to be poor; however, phoneme detection improved over the ensuing months, as noted by informal probes during mapping sessions. After 5 months experience with the BP+4 map, Child F could only discriminate syllabic patterns, not phonemes. When speech perception was tested using the Peabody Picture Vocabulary test, he obtained 22 out of 24 correct for the visual and auditory cues together, but only 2 out of 24 correct in the auditory-alone condition.

Seven months after receiving the implant, Child F was enrolled in a preschool program for children with hearing impairment that stressed auditory-aural modes of communication and included individual teaching sessions with a teacher of the deaf and with a speech therapist to improve listening skills and spoken language. A formal report written after 8 months in this program indicated that Child F's attention could only be gained by touching him or being in his line of vision and "it has been observed by all staff that after extensive listening training he still does not respond to his name during individual sessions or kindergarten time. (His) understanding of language . . . is based on context, routines, gestures and lip-reading." His speech was noted to be mostly unintelligible.

Because of his difficulty in using auditory signals, it was recommended that Child F be enrolled in a Total Communication Program that would incorporate manual communication. His speech perception scores at that time, determined using the PBK word lists, were 11% for phonemes, in the audition alone condition, 30% for phonemes in the audition plus visual condition, and 18% for phonemes in the visual alone (lip-reading) condition. At age 7 years, after 3 years of consistent implant use, it was noted that "He has shown no auditory progress over the last two years . . . while [he] is happy to wear the device, he shows no consistent awareness of sound." It should be noted that cochlear implant integrity testing (in the manner of Shallop, Kelsall, Caleffe-Schenk, & Ash, 1995) revealed normal device function.

Child F, 4.5 years after implantation and intensive aural–oral communication habilitation, continues to show speech perception only when he is able to access visual cues. Cochlear microphonics (but not otoacoustic emissions) are still present when the nonimplanted ear is tested (Figure 11–13). Picture vocabulary testing revealed 100% score for auditory plus visual mode, a 75% score for visual alone mode, and a score of 8% for auditory alone stimulus presentation. Speech perception was also tested using PBK words, and a phoneme score of 79% in the auditory plus visual condition, 75% for speech-reading alone, and 10% for auditory alone conditions.

The reasons why this child could not use electrical stimulation to access important cues for speech perception are not clear. Some children fail for reasons other than their "auditory capacity" with electrical stimulation. Those reasons include lack of auditory training, poor acceptance of the device, and poor parental follow-up. These were not issues for this child.

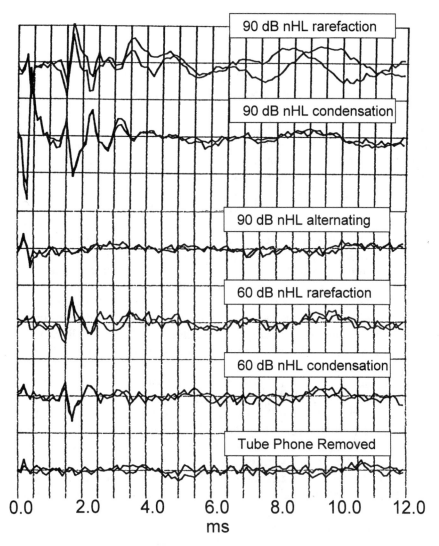

Figure 11–13. Cochlear microphonics recorded from the right (nonimplanted) ear when Child F was 8 years old. Cochlear microphonics are present for click stimuli at 60 dB nHL (95 dB peSPL) and above.

Some children with cochlear implants show more global language deficits. Child F's ability to utilize visual cues to reconstruct speech and linguistic elements would argue against a global language deficit in this child. The peripheral auditory system is implicated. Because his device was working properly, the need for using a BP+4 mapping strategy indicates the possibility of poor nerve survival. Unfortunately, this child cannot be distinguished from the others discussed here who obtained benefit from implantation based on history or any part of the test battery.

NEURAL RESPONSE TESTING

It was hypothesized that the improvements in speech perception noted in the first five patients was a result of enhanced temporal encoding and neural synchrony in response to electrical stimulation provided by the implant. Evoked potential recordings are utilized to assess neural synchrony and temporal coding. The electrically evoked compound action potential (ECAP) is the most direct measure of neural activity in patients with CI. These measurements were limited to intraoperative recordings or in patients with percutaneous plugs until recent advances in the Cochlear Corporation device (Gantz, Brown, & Abbas, 1994). The new Nucleus CI24M cochlear implant incorporates telemetry, known as Neural Response Telemetry (NRT), to measure the ECAP; see Abbas et al. (1999) for a detailed explanation. Briefly, NRT allows an evoked potential to be measured across a pair of electrodes along the array following stimulation of another site along the array. A subtraction technique is utilized to extract the ECAP from stimulus artifact by recording two tracings, one with and one without the removal of the neural potential using a forward masking paradigm. The ECAP is typically recorded as a negative peak (N1) followed by a positive peak (P2) with amplitude measured in μV.

Figures 11–14 through 11–17 plot the ECAP response for children A, B, C, and D who all received the Nucleus CI24M device. This testing was not performed in Child F, who was implanted with an earlier model cochlear implant. The response waveforms are presented as a function of current level. Although a neural response could not be elicited before implantation, a robust ECAP was recorded in response to electrical stimulation for each case. The response amplitude increases with increasing current level as would be expected of a functioning, neural system. The fact that an ECAP can be recorded in these patients indicates that electrical stimulation has restored some degree of neural synchrony and temporal encoding at the level of the auditory nerve.

Additional recordings of the electrically evoked ABR (EABR) in response to electrical stimulation were also obtained for Child B. Recording of the EABR provides documentation of synchronous neural activity in the auditory brain stem pathway in response to electrical stimulation, whereas the NRT only assesses the nerve. EABR tracings recorded at a current level set just below comfort level on electrode 20 are shown in Figure 11–18 for Child B. The presence of waves III and V is clearly indicated with latencies that are typical for a cochlear implant patient.

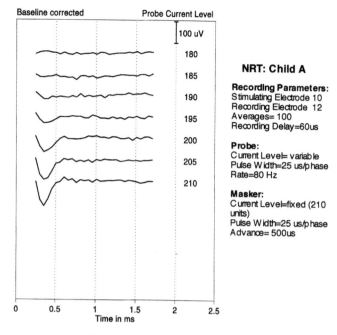

Figure 11–14. Electrical compound action potential recording for Child A.

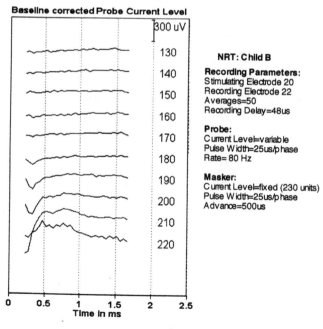

Figure 11–15. Electrical compound action potential recording for Child B.

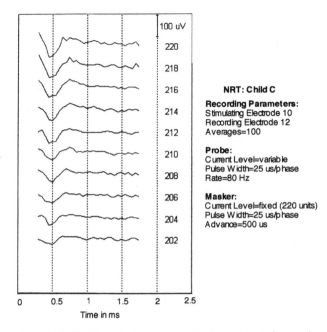

Figure 11–16. Electrical compound action potential recording for Child C.

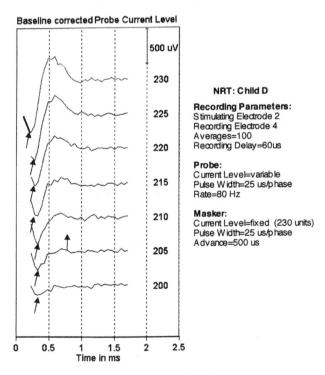

Figure 11–17. Electrical compound action potential recording for Child D.

228

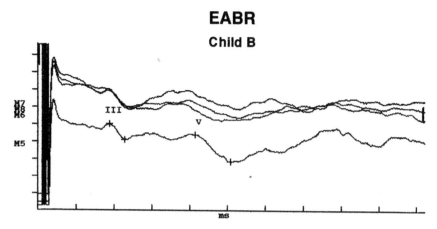

Figure 11–18. Electrical auditory brain stem response recording for Child B.

SUMMARY

These case studies demonstrate the potential for significant benefits from the use of cochlear implants in selected cases of auditory neuropathy. Electrical stimulation provided by a cochlear implant produced electrically evoked neural responses and significant improvement in speech perception abilities in five children with AN. The sixth case shows that improvement in speech perception is not guaranteed by cochlear implantation, however. The diagnosis of AN alone should not be grounds for an immediate referral for a cochlear implant evaluation. It is not clear what distinguished the poor implant user from the other patients in our series, nor do we have enough data to know how often to expect that the implant will not be successful in cases of AN. We do know, however, that some infants diagnosed with AN who initially presented behaviorally as deaf, show improved or fluctuating auditory responses with increasing age (Berlin, Goforth-Barter, St. John, & Hood, 1999). Although few, some patients have experienced some degree of benefit with conventional amplification in terms of speech perception (Cone-Wesson, Rance, & Sininger, Chapter 12 this volume; Rance et al., 1999). A trial period with conventional amplification is still recommended before implantation is considered.

All the children presented here were determined to be cochlear implant candidates under the current guidelines for implantation of children with cochlear hearing losses (i.e., they all demonstrated severe-to-profound hearing loss). Continued research in the areas of diagnosis, etiology, and pathophysiology of AN are needed before exploring the possibility of implanting patients having mild-to-severe audiometric thresholds in whom no benefit from conventional amplification is gained.

Indeed, the issue of amplification and cochlear implant use in patients with AN is still controversial and should be handled on an individual basis. The results of these cases are encouraging, however, and offer hope that electrical stimulation may improve access to auditory speech information in many patients with AN.

REFERENCES

Abbas, P. J., Brown, C. J., Shallop, J. K., Firszt, J. B., Hughes, M. L., Hong, S. H., & Staller, S. J. (1999). Summary of results using the Nucleus CI24M implant to record the electrically evoked compound action potential. *Ear and Hearing, 20,* 45–59.

Araki, S., Kawano, A., Seldon, L., Shepard, R. K., Funasaka, S., & Clark, G. M. (1998). Effects of chronic electrical stimulation on spiral ganglion neuron survival and size in deafened kittens. *The Laryngoscope, 108,* 687–695.

Berlin, C. I., Goforth-Barter, L., St. John, P., & Hood, L. (1999, February). *Auditory neuropathy: Three time courses after early identification.* Paper presented at the Twenty-Second Mid-Winter Meeting of the Association for Research in Otolaryngology, St. Petersburg, FL.

Berlin C. I., Hood L. J., Cecola P., Jackson D. F., & Szabo P. (1993). Does Type I afferent neuron dysfunction reveal itself through lack of efferent suppression? *Hearing Research, 65,* 40–50.

Cohen, N. L., Waltzman, S. B., Roland, J. T., Staller, S. J., & Hoffman, R. A. (1999). Early results using the CI24M in children. *American Journal of Otology, 20,* 198–204.

Gantz, B. J., Brown, C. J., & Abbas, P. J. (1994). Intraoperative measures of electrically evoked auditory nerve compound action potential. *American Journal of Otology, 15,* 137–144.

Gstoettner, W., Plenk, H. Jr., Franz, P., Hamzavi, J., Baumgartner, W., Czerny, C., & Ehrenberger, K. (1997). Cochlear implant deep insertion: Extent of insertion trauma. *Acta Otolaryngologica (Stockholm), 117,* 274–277.

Harrison, R. V. (1998) An animal model of auditory neuropathy. *Ear and Hearing, 19,* 355–361.

Haskins, H. (1949). *A phonetically balanced test of speech discrimination for children.* Unpublished master's thesis, Northwestern University, Evanston, IL.

Ling, D. (1978). Speech development in hearing-impaired children. *Journal of Communication Disorders, 11,* 119–124.

McKay, C. M., McDermott, H. J., Vandali, A. E., & Clark, G. M. (1992). A comparison of speech perception of cochlear implantees using the spectral maximum sound processor (SMSP) and the MSP (MULTIPEAK) processor. *Acta Otolaryngologica (Stockholm), 112,* 752–761.

Mitchell, A., Miller, J. M., Finger, P. A., Heller, J. W., Raphael, Y., & Altschuler, R. A. (1997). Effects of chronic high-rate electrical stimulation on the cochlea and eighth nerve in the deafened guinea pig. *Hearing Research, 105,* 30–43.

Miyamoto, R. T., Kirk, K. I., Svirsky, M. A., & Sehgal, S. T. (1999). Communication skills in pediatric cochlear implant recipients. *Acta Otolaryngologica (Stockholm), 119,* 219–224.

Moog, J. S., & Geers, A. E. (1990). *Early speech perception test.* St. Louis, MO: Central Institute for the Deaf.

O'Donoghue, G. M., Nikolopoulos, T. P., Archbold, S. M., & Tait, M. (1998). Speech perception in children after cochlear implantation. *American Journal of Otology, 19,* 762–767.

O'Leary, M. J., Fayad, J., House, W. F., & Linthicum, F. H. Jr. (1991). Electrode insertion trauma in cochlear implantation. *Annals of Otology, Rhinology and Laryngology, 100,* 695–699.

O'Leary, S. J., Mitchell, T. E., Gibson, W. P., & Sanli, H. (in press). Abnormal positive potentials in round window electrocochleography. *American Journal of Otology.*

Rance, G., Beer, D. E., Cone-Wesson, B., Shepherd, R. K., Dowell, R. C., King, A. M., Rickards, F. W., & Clark, G. M. (1999) Clinical findings in a group of infants and young children with auditory neuropathy. *Ear and Hearing, 20,* 238–252.

Seewald, R. C., Ross, M., & Spiro, M. K. (1985). Selecting amplification characteristics for young hearing-impaired children. *Ear and Hearing, 6,* 48–53.

Shallop, J. K., Kelsall, D. C., Caleffe-Schenk, N., & Ash, K. R. (1995). Application of averaged voltages in the management of cochlear implant patients. *Annals of Otology, Rhinology and Laryngology Supplement, 166,* 228–230.

Shannon, R. V. (1993) Quantitative comparison of electrically and acoustically evoked auditory perception: Implications for location of perceptual mechanisms. *Progress in Brain Research, 97,* 261–269.

Sininger, Y. S., Trautwein, P. G., Shallop, J. K., Fabry, L. B., & Starr, A. (1999, February). *Electrical activation of the auditory nerve in patients with auditory neuropathy.* Paper presented at the Twenty-Second Annual Association for Research in Otolaryngology Mid-Winter Meeting, St. Petersburg, FL.

Skinner, M. W., Clark, G. M., Whitford, L. A., Seligman, P. M., & Staller, S. J. (1994). Evaluation of a new spectral peak coding strategy for the Nucleus 22 cochlear implant system. *American Journal of Otology, 15,* 15–27.

Stein, L., Tremblay, K., Pasternak, J., Banerjee, S., Lindemann, K., & Krauss, N. (1996). Brainstem abnormalities in neonates with normal otoacoustic emissions. *Seminars in Hearing, 17,* 197–213.

Tramell, J., & Owens, S. (1977). *Test of Auditory Comprehension.* North Hollywood, CA: Foreworks Publishing.

Trautwein, P. G., Sininger, Y. S., & Nelson, R. (2000). Cochlear implantation of auditory neuropathy. *Journal of the American Academy of Audiology, 11,* 309–315.

Zeng, F.-G., Oba, S., Garde, S., Sininger, Y., & Starr, A. (1999). Temporal processing impairment in auditory neuropathy. *NeuroReport, 10,* 3429–3435.

Zhou, R., Abbas, P. J., & Assouline, J. S. (1995). Electrically evoked auditory brainstem response in myelin-deficient mice. *Hearing Research, 88,* 98–106.

Zhou, R., Assouline, J. G., Abbas, P. J., Messing, A., & Gantz, B. J. (1995). Anatomical and physiological measures of auditory system in mice with peripheral myelin deficiency. *Hearing Research, 88,* 87–97.

Amplification and Rehabilitation Strategies for Patients With Auditory Neuropathy

Barbara Cone-Wesson, Gary Rance, and Yvonne Sininger

The lack of knowledge about the exact pathology of auditory neuropathy type hearing loss and a lack of knowledge about the exact nature of the hearing disability has resulted in considerable controversy regarding whether hearing devices (hearing aids, personal radio-frequency [FM] units, or cochlear implants) should be used and the types of (re)habilitation that should accompany the provision of such devices. Some children with severe-to-profound hearing loss and auditory neuropathy have received cochlear implants, and their case histories and the results of this treatment are summarized in Chapter 11 by Trautwein et al. This chapter will provide current data regarding the use of amplification in children with auditory neuropathy hearing loss. The aural-oral and visual-manual approaches to language development among infants and children with auditory neuropathy hearing loss will also be reviewed. We will integrate what is known about psychophysical performance and speech perception abilities in patients with this hearing disorder and suggest approaches to hearing aid fitting that are based on these findings.

PSYCHOACOUSTICS AND SPEECH PERCEPTION ABILITIES

Zeng, Oba, Garde, Sininger, and Starr (1999) assessed patients with auditory neuropathy using sophisticated psychophysical tests to understand the basic hearing deficits underlying the speech understanding disability.

The subjects' temporal processing abilities were assessed in three detection tasks: first, for brief tones (temporal integration); second, for a silent period embedded in a noise burst (gap detection); and third, for fluctuations in level of a steady-state noise (modulation transfer function). Gap detection and the modulation transfer functions were abnormal in patients with auditory neuropathy. These findings (reported in detail in Chapter 8) relate the electrophysiologic findings in auditory neuropathy, specifically, a lack of neural synchrony resulting in absent short-latency evoked potentials, to basic psychophysical abilities underlying speech sound understanding. The lack of neural synchrony is hypothesized to cause "a [time] smeared internal representation of a physical stimulus" (Zeng et al., 1999, p. 3434).

Speech understanding is contingent on the processing of subtle temporal cues in the signal. Such skills would be reflected in a high degree of sensitivity for short gaps and amplitude modulations. Zeng et al. (1999) proposed that a special type of speech processing hearing aid is needed for people with auditory neuropathy. In addition to amplifying sounds to make them audible, they suggested that a hearing aid "should compensate for the impaired temporal processing at suprathreshold levels." One such approach would be a speech-processing-type hearing aid that emphasized transient sounds. As a first approximation to this, hearing aids with a high-frequency emphasis might serve to emphasize the high-frequency transient speech sounds, in particular, the high-frequency consonants.

Starr and colleagues' thorough electrophysiologic and psychoacoustic description of one patient with a neuropathic type degenerative hearing loss (Starr et al., 1991) also points to the need for hearing devices that overcome the effect of temporal dysynchrony on speech understanding. Conventional amplification appeared to be of no benefit to speech understanding for this young woman, who developed moderate hearing loss and speech perception disability at about 9 years of age. The larger group of patients with auditory neuropathy described by Starr, Picton, Sininger, Hood, and Berlin (1996) had speech perception scores that ranged from 0 to 92%. None of the subjects was reported to obtain benefit from conventional amplification; however, aided versus unaided speech perception scores were not reported.

The hallmark of auditory neuropathy is very poor speech perception, particularly in light of pure tone sensitivity. There are, however, individuals with auditory neuropathy who show speech perception abilities, although impaired, similar to those of individuals with the same degree of sensorineural hearing loss, at least when tested at suprathreshold levels. Performance-intensity functions in auditory neuropathy hearing loss have not been shown, and therefore it is not known whether performance would decrease dramatically with increasing presentation level, as in the rollover typical of other retrocochlear losses or whether only a slight decrease or saturating function might be seen. Because the desired outcome of amplification is improved speech perception, and if speech perception can be shown to increase with sound presentation level, it would appear that knowledge of the performance-intensity function may be helpful for determining hearing aid benefit.

AMPLIFICATION

Among the adults studied by Starr et al. (1996) amplification was of no benefit, and in some cases led to "detrimental effects." Because of this report, there has existed a reluctance to recommend hearing aids for infants and children affected by auditory neuropathy (Berlin, 1999; Doyle, Sininger, & Starr, 1998).

Despite the presence of "normal" outer hair cell (OHC) function, at least as evidenced by the presence of evoked otoacoustic emissions (OAEs), cochlear microphonics (CMs), or both, amplification can provide useful hearing to some children with auditory neuropathy. Rance et al. (1999) were the first to show that approximately 50% of affected children benefit from amplification. Hearing aid benefit was investigated in eight children who were able to complete formal speech perception testing in both unaided and aided conditions. Four of the eight subjects showed significantly higher scores in the aided condition and, in fact, performed at levels expected for children with comparable degrees of sensorineural hearing loss. The other four subjects, however, did not score at significant levels in either the unaided or aided testing conditions. In these children, the lack of aided benefit did not appear to be related to their behavioral hearing levels. Two children presented with profound hearing loss, whereas two had unaided thresholds in only the mild-to-moderate range. Overall, the results from the Rance et al. series indicated that it was not possible to predict from either the pure-tone audiogram or the unaided speech perception scores which children would benefit from amplification.

A sample of 29 children followed at the House Ear Institute revealed that 14 (52%) are "past users" or "nonusers" of hearing aids, suggesting no benefit. Of the patients who were deemed to have received some useful aided hearing, three (10%) showed fair-to-good benefit as evidenced by improvement in both pure-tone thresholds and speech perception in the aided mode. It should be noted that these three patients have lost their OAEs (see Chapter 2 by Sininger and Oba), and it is possible that they now have a sensory component to their hearing loss. Five of those patients considered as showing benefit demonstrated some improvement in aided thresholds without dramatic increase in speech perception (17% of total showed fair improvement). Among the remainder of patients are those who are very young or difficult to test. Some of these patients may become nonusers but for the present they are using amplification. For each of the children in this later group, we have anecdotal reports from parents, educators, or both that they are consistent users, and the parents and teachers of these children have reported some aided benefit.

Results from the House Ear Institute are similar to the findings from the Melbourne series (Rance et al., 1999), showing no useful aided hearing in approximately 50% of the sample. In these examples, benefit of amplification was quantified by use of speech perception test scores, whereas previously published reports regarding the use of amplification with auditory neuropathy have often been based on the patient's own impressions of the hearing aids, rather than a quantitative measure.

The presence of OAEs or CMs in patients with auditory neuropathy suggests that the cochlea has a normal complement of OHCs, the cells that provide the exquisite sensitivity and tuning that is the hallmark of the normal cochlea. Likewise, it is damage or loss of OHCs that is the underlying pathology of most sensory hearing loss of moderate degree or less. In auditory neuropathy, there appears to be a disconnection between the integrity of the OHCs and their functional effects. It is not surprising that some patients with auditory neuropathy have functional hearing disabilities similar to those of patients with sensory losses, who, having lost a complement of outer hair cells, have absent OAEs and acoustic reflexes, pure-tone threshold impairment, and poor speech perception.

There has been some suggestion that amplification should not be used for children with auditory neuropathy or, if hearing aids are tried, that fittings should be unilateral and conservative in terms of gain. Hood (1998) recommended:

> high quality, low gain, wide dynamic range compression hearing aids. This approach is intended to minimize any deleterious effects of amplification on otoacoustic emissions until the importance of maintaining otoacoustic emissions in these patients is better understood ... If hearing aids are tried, frequent monitoring of otoacoustic emissions for either temporary or permanent effects on OAEs should be part of the management program. (p. 10)

Because it has now been shown that OAEs may deteriorate in some children with auditory neuropathy (while the cochlear microphonic, CM, is maintained; Deltenre et al., 1999; Rance et al., 1999) without any change in pure-tone sensitivity, there may be considerable risk that children with auditory neuropathy have inadequate amplification for their hearing needs. The reasoning behind the Hood methodology appears to be the sparing of OHCs by preventing temporary or permanent threshold shift owing to noise exposure from hearing aids. It is not clear, however, that the outer hair cells that generate the OAEs or CMs provide any functional benefit in terms of sensitivity or frequency discrimination in those who have auditory neuropathy.

Hearing aids can cause significant noise exposure and permanent threshold shift in children with sensorineural hearing loss (Macrae, 1991, 1994, 1995). Macrae (1995) measured the permanent threshold shift experienced by eight children using monaurally fit power hearing aids for 6 to 8 years for their moderate to moderately severe hearing losses. Permanent threshold shift was demonstrated in all cases, with average shifts of 15 to 20 dB after 8 years of use. The shift in threshold over time showed an asymptotic function, in accordance with a model of temporary threshold shift (Macrae, 1995). Macrae showed that fitting with a real ear insertion response recommended by National Acoustics Laboratory (Australia) will prevent temporary and permanent threshold shift, except for those children who use high gain amplification, such as for profound losses, that is, with average hearing losses $\geq$ 100 dB HL (Macrae, 1995). The benefit of hearing sound, especially speech, must be weighed against the possibility of permanent threshold shift of up to 20 dB. This is the risk–benefit ratio calculated for any child who needs amplification. Hood (1998) suggested that if more powerful hearing aids are recommended for children with auditory neuropathy, they should be worn for limited time periods or in only one ear, so that one ear is spared the risk of permanent threshold shift.

The first five children with auditory neuropathy identified by the Melbourne group were amplified conservatively in the initial period to reduce the possibility of cochlear insult. Hearing aids were fit binaurally with gain and maximum power output settings at levels appropriate for mild hearing loss. In each of these cases, anecdotal reports at the end of 6 months consistent aid use from parents and "teachers of the deaf" indicated little or no sound detection. When these children were subsequently fitted in accordance with their behavioral audiograms using the National Acoustics Laboratory (Australia) rules, none showed tolerance problems or significant threshold shift, and four of the five children demonstrated rapid improvements in speech awareness and general responsiveness.

In an attempt to identify factors relevant to the treatment and habilitation of children with auditory neuropathy (such as age of identification, provision of amplification, and education strategy), we have reviewed the histories of affected children from the University of Melbourne, School of Audiology clinic. These results, along with the speech perception scores, are found in Table 12–1. Ten of 17 children had their hearing loss identified by 6 months of age, likely owing to the fact that the Victorian Infant Hearing Screening Program mandated an auditory brain stem response (ABR) hearing screening test for all children with risk factors for hearing loss, including those who were cared for in a newborn intensive care unit. It is not surprising that Case 5 had late detection of hearing problems because

Table 12–1. Summary of factors relevant to auditory neuropathy.

Case	Age at Diagnosis (months)	3 Freq Average	Age Aided (Months)	History with Amplification	Age in Years of (Aided PBK)	PBK Score (%)	Habilitation History
1	3	38	5	Uses hearing aids consistently.	3	39	Oral preschool for deaf & h-h.[a] Now in oral program at primary school for deaf and h-h.
2	5	40	NA	NA	5	CNA	Child has cerebral palsy and receives physical therapy for spasticity.
3	2	40	6	Uses hearing aids consistently.	4	57	Parent advisor service.[b]
4	6	40	NA			NA	Multiply disabled.
5	28	42	33	Inconsistent user for 9 months; good user from 3.5 yrs	7	96	Oral preschool for deaf and h-h. Now mainstreamed with teacher aid support.
6	1	45	24	Uses hearing aids consistently.	4	4	Total communication primary school program.
7[c]	1	20	NA				
7	60	50	60	Uses hearing aids consistently.	6	85	Mainstream at primary school, has teacher of deaf support for 1 hour/day.
8	14	53	16	Uses hearing aids consistently.	4	43	Child has moved interstate. Information not available.
9	8	55	12	Used hearing aids as an infant. Not a consistent user now.	4	6	Oral preschool for deaf and h-h. Now in TC primary school program.
10	4	60	6	Uses hearing aids consistently.	5	85	Oral preschool for the deaf and h-h. Oral program at primary school for deaf and h-h.
11	21	75	4	Uses hearing aids consistently.	4	70	Oral preschool for deaf and h-h. Integrated into local primary school.

Table 12–1. (continued)

Case	Age at Diagnosis (months)	3 Freq Average	Age Aided (Months)	History with Amplification	Age in Years of (Aided PBK)	PBK Score (%)	Habilitation History
12	12	85	18	Uses hearing aids consistently.	4	6	In-home instruction in sign language (Auslan) for parents and child.
13	1	98	5	Uses hearing aids consistently.	5	59	In-home instruction in sign language (Auslan). Signing primary school.
14	8	100	10	Uses hearing aids consistently. Being considered for cochlear implant.	2.5	51	In-home instruction in sign language (Auslan) for parents and child, now in oral program at preschool for deaf and h-h.
15	8	118	14	Used hearing aids consistently. Has used a cochlear implant consistently since 3.5 years.	8	8	Oral preschool for deaf and h-h. Until recently in oral program at primary school for deaf and h-h but has now transferred to signing stream.
16	18	120	19	Used hearing aids consistently. Now uses a cochlear implant inconsistently.	5	9: 77 with CI	Local primary school with aid support.
17	1	>120	6	Hearing aids used inconsistently. Received CI at age 4 but facial nerve stimulation prevents usage.	4	6	Oral preschool for deaf and h-h. Now uses Auslan at home and school.

Note. [a]"Special school for deaf and hard of hearing children (not mainstreamed).
[b]"Parent Advisor Service" provides sign language instruction for deaf children and their families along with other counselling, educational, and social programs.
[c]This child contracted meningitis at age 5 years, with subsequent drop in hearing thresholds. He did not use amplification prior to the loss of pure-tone sensitivity.
Auslan = Australian Sign Language; CI = cochlear implant; h-h = hard of hearing.

this child had none of the conventional risk factors for hearing loss, had a fluctuating mild-moderate hearing loss, and at times had normal speech perception.

An auditory–oral education strategy was initially employed with 14 of the 17 children. Four of these children subsequently shifted (after approximately 9 to 12 months) to an educational approach emphasizing visual communication (sign language) after they had failed to progress auditorally. Another child (Case 15) changed from an oral to a signing strategy at the age of 9 years.

Three children were educated using sign language from the time of their diagnosis. In two of the cases, the child lived in an isolated region where only sign-based education strategies were available. In the other, it was the choice of the parents to pursue the signing option.

Age of detection and consistent hearing aid use did not appear to be factors determining speech perception benefit in this sample of children, nor was habilitation strategy. There was a trend toward poorer speech perception scores in the children educated in signing settings, but this is most likely a reflection of the inherent processing abilities of each child rather than the educational strategy; that is, the children whose speech perception was most disabled by the auditory neuropathy were those who could not cope with audition-based education systems and who moved to visual-based programs where they could succeed more readily.

SPEECH AND LANGUAGE DEVELOPMENT FOR THE CHILD WITH AUDITORY NEUROPATHY

As for any infant or child with a hearing loss, intervention and enrichment strategies for the development of language will be at a priority. The debate concerning "oral" versus "manual" methods of language learning cannot be escaped in the arena of language facilitation for the child with congenital auditory neuropathy type hearing loss. For at least the past 250 years, there have been philosophical and even religious debates about the superiority of either manualism or oralism for communication with and among persons who are deaf or who have a hearing loss (Rée, 1999). Oralism was advocated as a language learning method almost two centuries before any kind of amplification or hearing prosthetics were available. Likewise, manualism, or sign language, has long been regarded by many as the native and superior language for those who do not have hearing, even when hearing prosthetics are an option.

In this chapter, evidence is presented that amplification can be of benefit to some children with auditory neuropathy, and in another (see Trautwein et al., Chapter 11), case studies are presented in which benefit from cochlear implantation is demonstrated. Further research is needed to understand if there are any predisposing factors that may be predictive of benefit from one type of hearing prosthetic over another. The range of speech and language outcomes vary dramatically even for children with sensory loss of similar degree and with similar amplification or implantation histories. This will be no different for children with auditory neuropathy.

The principles of early intervention and habilitation of speech and language for the child with auditory neuropathy are similar to those for the child with sensorineural hearing loss. Families need nonbiased information about and access to resources that will guide their decision as to which communication and language approach, educational method, and service options best fit their own situation (Mertens, Sass-Lehrer, & Scott-Olson, 2000).

Cued Speech

Because little is known about the perceptual abilities in the child with auditory neuropathy and because the auditory signal is disrupted to different degrees, visual modes of communication would appear to be a logical choice to supplement auditory presentation of spoken language in some cases. One method of visual support of spoken language is cued speech. Cued speech is a method for providing a manual-visual aid to lipreading. Cued speech was developed by Cornett (1967) as a manual representation of phonologic cues that are used simultaneously with oral speech. The phonologic representations are depicted by a series of handshapes that are made in various positions at the speaker's mouth or at the level of the larynx. These give cues to vowel or consonant sounds (or their manner of production) that are difficult or ambiguous to perceive from lipreading alone, allowing the receiver to simultaneously detect sounds that are visually available via speech reading as well as those sounds that are not visualized but indicated by the cueing. Cued speech is a visual aid to supplement or may even enhance speech perception from lipreading and audition. On a practical basis, it is similar to providing a visual sign or symbol for sounds or words that cannot be perceived by audition alone. On a theoretical level, because the cues are for phonologic rather than orthographic (as for finger spelling) representation of speech, it has been suggested that cued speech can aid in the development of phonologic representation of language for children who are deaf or hard of hearing (Charlier, 1992). Cued speech has been used in conjunction with oral–aural methods of language development, with total communication and with Signed French.[1]

---

[1] "Signed French is expressed in a linear manner, simultaneously speaking audibly and taking vocabulary from Sign Language. Signed words are thus accompanied by spoken words without any modification of the grammatical structure of the French language" (Charlier, 1992, p. 334).

Particular advantages of cued speech as a supplement to aural–oral methods are that the syntax of the spoken English, and the phonologic structure of the language is conveyed. Another is that the cueing system may be learned more rapidly by hearing parents than a complete sign language, such as American Sign Language or Auslan (Australian Sign Language), because it is based on the hearing person's native language. A disadvantage is that cued speech resources, such as instruction in cued speech, and persons trained as "transliterators" for the child in the classroom, may be very limited (Reamy & Brackett, 1999).

Berlin and colleagues (personal communication, 1999) have advocated the use of cued speech as a communication mode to facilitate language learning in children with auditory neuropathy, which they term "auditory dysynchrony." They provided anecdotal data as well as some parent testimonial concerning the success of cued speech as a communication mode for children with auditory neuropathy–dysynchrony.

Other Methods of Visually Supported Spoken Language

Total Communication, Sim-Com (Simultaneous Communication), and manually coded English are other methods in which both audible speech and visual signs are presented to ensure that a child has access to any means possible for learning language. Total Communication was first advocated as a method to link aural–oral and manual communication systems. Presently, total communication methods utilize elements of sign language with an English-based syntax, and spoken language together, although recognizing that in certain situations, American Sign Language alone or spoken English alone may be preferable (Reamy & Brackett, 1999). The Sim-Com educational strategy combines the use of sign and speech, with the purpose of conveying language and communicating by "every available means" (Tye-Murray, 1998, p. 394). Manually coded English presents language visually through signs, together with speech, using English syntax, and includes manual signs for morphemic word endings. Some manifestations of this strategy are referred to as Signed English, Seeing Essential English, Signing Exact English, and Linguistics of Visual English (Tye-Murray, 1998). The advantage of a visually supported spoken language is that if the child cannot *hear* the spoken language, there is a signing (manual–visual) system that conveys meaning. The disadvantage is that signed languages, such as American Sign Language, have their own syntax and are complete language systems that may be degraded rather than enhanced by the simultaneous presentation of spoken English. It is the case, however, that the vast majority of specialized educational programs for children with hearing loss utilize some type of Total Communication or Sim-Com system (Meadow-Orlans, 2000).

Language conveys culture, and it is an abiding principle that a child should be brought up in the culture and language system of the parent. For the child with hearing loss, whether sensory, neural, or a combination of both, the language of the parent(s) is most often spoken language. Hearing parents of children who are deaf or who have significant auditory problems, such as in auditory neuropathy, can also be given the opportunity to learn sign language to communicate with their child. A recent case study (Spencer, 2000) documents the success of one family in which hearing parents supported the use of American Sign Language, Deaf Culture, spoken language and hearing (with a cochlear implant) for their deaf child.

CASE STUDY

Chapter 11 included six cases of children in whom no benefit was found using amplification and for whom a cochlear implant was recommended. The following case provides an example of a young child who, despite presenting with severe-to-profound hearing loss, showed significant speech perception improvements when wearing conventionally fitted hearing aids.

History and Initial Test Results

The child in question had a normal birth history, and there were no risk factors for hearing loss. The infant (Y) had failed a behavioral hearing screening test carried out at 8 months of age, and the parents had been concerned about a lack of responsiveness to sound in the environment from the age of 6 months. Within 1 month of failing the distraction test, Y had undergone an audiologic evaluation including behavioral hearing tests, tympanometry, OAEs, ABRs, and steady-state evoked potential (SSEP) tests.

The results of that evaluation showed no aural–palpebral reflexes to loud sound. A type A tympanogram was found in the right ear and a type B in the left ear (with otoscopic evidence of middle ear effusion). Distortion-product otoacoustic emissions (DPOAEs) were present for the right ear but not the left. ABR showed CMs present for both ears with 70 dB nHL clicks, but no action potential (AP) or wave V was evident for either ear at levels up to 90 dB nHL for the left ear and 70 dB nHL for the right ear. Later testing showed no ABR waveforms in either ear to clicks at 90 dB nHL.

Steady-state evoked potentials were tested using tones modulated at 90 Hz (Rance, Richards, Cohen, DeVidi, & Clark, 1995). Using regression equations developed from behavioral and SSEP threshold data from infants, children, and adults with sensory impairment (Rance et al., 1995), the SSEP results in this patient would have been consistent with a moderate-to-severe loss for the right ear and a severe-to-profound loss for the left ear. However, analyses of SSEP data from a group of children with auditory neuropathy showed that SSEP thresholds were generally discrepant from behavioral thresholds (Rance et al., 1999).

Amplification

Y was fitted binaurally within 2 weeks of the audiologic evaluation with mild gain hearing aids. It was noted that Y did not have any noticeable change in behavior when wearing the instruments. The audiologist monitored aid use on a biweekly basis for several months and gradually increased the gain to levels appropriate for a child with sensorineural hearing loss of moderate-to-severe degree. Y remained unresponsive to sound.

Because Y was not responding to the amplified signal, the parents investigated whether cochlear implantation would be beneficial. As part of that evaluation, extratympanic electrocochleography was carried out under general anesthesia, as was a repeated SSEP test. CM responses were evident in response to unipolar clicks at 90 dB nHL for both ears; SSEP results were unchanged for the left ear, but indicated thresholds 25 dB poorer for the right ear (thresholds changed from 75 dB HL previously to 100 dB HL). It was at this time, when Y was 13 months old, that reliable thresholds were obtained using visual reinforcement audiometry (VRA) procedures. The audiogram shown in Figure 12–1 indicated a severe-to-profound hearing loss for the better ear. Acoustic reflexes were absent for both ipsilateral and contralateral stimulation, although the left ear tympanogram still indicated lower than normal admittance. Subsequent VRA tests completed over the next few weeks confirmed and extended the initial results, indicating a symmetrical severe-to-profound impairment for both ears. Based on this behavioral information, the gain of the hearing aids was increased, and aided sound-field thresholds were obtained within the speech spectrum (Figure 12–2). It was also noted that Y showed a noticeable alerting to voices, once the amplification gain was increased.

Over the next few months, Y continued to show an increase in responsiveness when wearing the hearing aids, and changes were documented using the meaningful auditory integration (Robbins et al., 1991). Y's scores on this inventory improved from 5 out of 40 items after 1 month of hearing aid use to 16 out of 40 items after 6 months of high gain hearing aid use. Y's candidacy for a cochlear implant was still at issue, but with the noticeable improvement obtained with conventional amplification, the parents were counseled to persist with hearing aids until it was possible to undertake measures of speech perception.

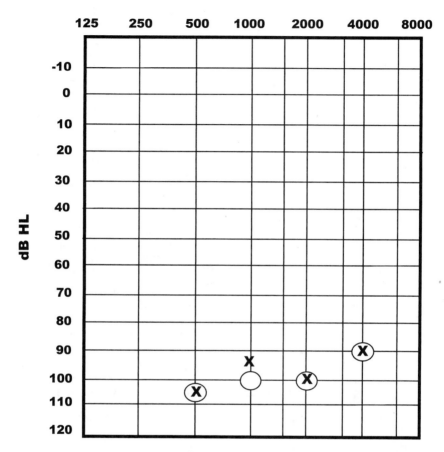

Figure 12–1. Pure-tone audiogram obtained using visual reinforcement audiometry procedures under earphones when Y was 13 months old. Tympanometry showed low immittance for the left ear but was within normal limits for the right ear.

Habilitation

In addition to having the hearing loss diagnosed by 8 months of age and hearing aids fit shortly thereafter, Y was enrolled in a total communication program. Y's parents learned sign language and also used voice with signs together in a consistent manner. At age 2.5 years, Y started using a personal FM system in addition to consistent use of hearing aids. At 2 years 9 months of age, Y was reevaluated with behavioral hearing tests and formal speech perception assessments. A pure-tone audiogram was obtained using play procedures, which showed a bilateral profound loss for both

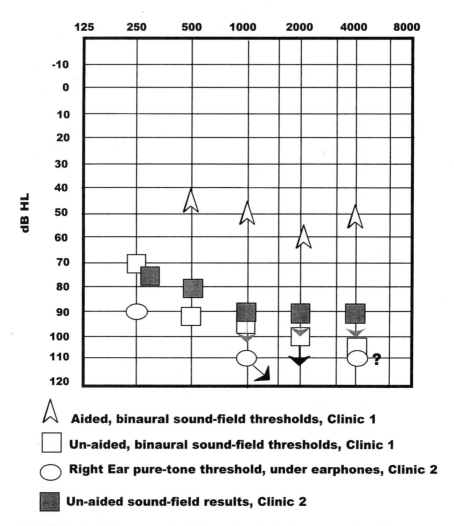

Figure 12–2. Audiogram and aided results obtained using visual reinforcement audiometry when Y was 14–15 months and hearing aid gain had been increased to provide gain for a severe-to-profound hearing loss. Two different audiology clinics were working collaboratively to obtain results and to document benefit from amplification.

ears, with slightly poorer thresholds in the low frequencies compared to the high frequencies. Informal observation of speech and language showed that Y used signs with voice to communicate and that speech production, which included two and three word phrases, was reasonably intelligible to an unfamiliar listener. Open-set speech perception was evaluated using phonetically balanced kindergarten word lists in the aided and unaided, audition-alone conditions. Y scored at chance levels (4%) when unaided, but obtained a phoneme score of 47% and a word score of 2 out of 25 (8%) when binaurally aided. Speech perception testing repeated 1 year later showed similar results with an aided phoneme score of 52% and word score of 12%. These scores are slightly poorer than those of the average child who uses a cochlear implant to hear (Dowell et al., 2000). As such, despite the fact (or because of the fact) that Y makes good use of residual hearing, implantation has been recommended, and Y is scheduled to receive the device in the near future.

SUMMARY AND CONCLUSIONS

The underlying pathophysiology of auditory neuropathy is yet undetermined, and it appears that several different sites of lesion may produce the same kind of functional result, specifically, impairment of pure-tone sensitivity and speech perception that is poorer than normal. More research needs to be completed concerning the perceptual effects of auditory neuropathy, and a nosology based on perceptual classification may help to guide treatment strategies.

Amplifying sound appears to benefit only 50% of the children who have auditory neuropathy. That benefit has been documented with both anecdotal reports and speech perception tests. Prolonged exposure to high levels of sound can cause hearing loss, but by using an algorithmic approach to hearing aid fitting, and real-ear measures to verify the parameters of the hearing aid, permanent threshold shift may be avoided in all but those with severe-to-profound hearing loss. Because the loss of OAEs can occur without amplification (Deltenre, 1999), and does not appear to affect pure-tone sensitivity or other perceptions, monitoring the effects of noise exposure with OAEs may be misleading. The aim of the hearing aid fitting should be to make speech audible. The use of a monaural amplification strategy is a conservative approach to this issue and may suit the needs of some children and their families. Experimental results from psychoacoustic testing (Zeng et al., 1999) suggest that speech processing strategies to improve transient perception (consonants) may be of benefit; whether this can be achieved with a high-frequency-emphasis-type hearing aid remains to be tested. Because it has been documented that patients with auditory neuropathy may also have a significantly poorer speech perception in background noise, even when pure-tone thresholds are normal (Kraus et al., 2000; Chapter 1 of this volume), directional microphones or the use of personal FM systems to improve the signal-to-noise ratio should be considered.

Working to develop language and speech in the child with auditory neuropathy is often more challenging than the same task in a child with sensory hearing loss. An aural–oral speech and language approach that may be appropriate for a child with sensory loss will not be effective for the child with auditory neuropathy, and a visual-manual support system such as Cued Speech, Total Communication, Sim-Com, or other signed English systems should be encouraged for children with auditory neuropathy.

Acknowledgments: The authors acknowledge contributions to this chapter by Dr. Charles Berlin (sections on cued speech). Ms. Sandy Oba contributed to the acquisition and reporting of data from the House Ear Institute. Ms. Alison King of Australian Hearing provided information regarding amplification for the Melbourne data. Portions of this work were supported by the National Institute on Deafness and Other Communicative Disorders Grant No. DC02618 (Sininger) and the Hearing Research Fund of the Bionic Ear Institute, and the University of Melbourne (Cone-Wesson and Rance).

REFERENCES

Berlin, C. I. (1999). Auditory neuropathy: Using OAEs and ABRs from screening to management. *Seminars in Hearing, 20,* 307–315.

Charlier, B. L. (1992). Complete signed and cued French. *American Annals of the Deaf, 137,* 331–337.

Cornett, O. (1967). Cued speech. *American Annals of the Deaf, 112,* 3–13.

Deltenre, P., Mansbach, A. L., Bozet, C., Christiaens, F., Barthelmy, P., Paulissen, D., & Renglet, T. (1999). Auditory neuropathy with preserved cochlear microphonics and secondary loss of otoacoustic emissions. *Audiology, 38,* 187–195.

Dowell, R. C. (2000, June). Speech perception in children using multichannel cochlear implants: Long-term results and predictive factors. *Proceedings of the Fifth European Symposium on Paediatric Cochlear Implantation,* Antwerp, Belgium.

Doyle, K. J., Sininger, Y. S., & Starr, A. (1998). Auditory neuropathy in childhood. *The Laryngoscope, 108,* 1374–1377.

Hood, L. J. (1998). Auditory neuropathy: What is it and what can we do about it. *The Hearing Journal, 51,* 10–18.

Kraus, N., Bradlow, A. R., Cheatham, J., Cunningham, C. D., King, D. B., Koch, T. G., Nicol, T. J., McGee, L. K., Stein, L. K., & Wright, B. A. (2000). Consequences of neural asynchrony: A case of auditory neuropathy. *Journal of the Association for Research in Otolaryngology, 1,* 33–45.

Macrae, J. H. (1991). Permanent threshold shift associated with overamplification by hearing aids. *Journal of Speech and Hearing Research, 34,* 403–414.

Macrae, J. H. (1994). Prediction of asymptotic threshold shift caused by hearing aid use. *Journal of Speech and Hearing Research, 37,* 227–237.

Maccrae, J. H. (1995). Temporary and permanent threshold shift caused by hearing aid use. *Journal of Speech and Hearing Research, 38,* 949–959.

Meadow-Orlans, K. P. (2000). Deafness and social change: Ruminations of a retiring researcher. In P. E. Spencer, C. J. Erting, & M. Marschark (Eds.), *The deaf child in the family and at school, Essays in honor of Kathryn P. Meadow-Orlans.* London: Lawrence Erlbaum Associates.

Mertens, D. M., Sass-Lehrer, M., & Scott-Olson, K. (2000). Sensitivity in family-professional relationship: Parental experiences in families with young deaf and hard of hearing children. In P. E. Spencer, C. J. Erting, & M. Marschark (Eds.), *The deaf child in the family and at school, Essays in honor of Kathryn P. Meadow-Orlans.* London: Lawrence Erlbaum Associates.

Rance, G., Rickards, F. W., Cohen, L. T., De Vidi, S., & Clark, G. M. (1995). The automated prediction of hearing thresholds in sleeping subjects using auditory steady-state evoked potentials. *Ear and Hearing, 16,* 499–507.

Rance G., Beer D. E., Cone-Wesson, B., Shepherd, R. K., Dowell, R. C., King, A. M., Rickards, F. W., & Clark, G. M. (1999). Clinical findings for a group of infants and young children with auditory neuropathy. *Ear and Hearing, 20,* 238–252.

Rée, J. (1999). *I see a voice: A philosophical history of language, deafness and the senses.* London: HarperCollins.

Reamy, C. E., & Brackett, D. (1999). Communication methodologies. *Otolaryngologic Clinics of North America, 32,* 1103–1116.

Robbins, A. M., Renshaw, J. J., & Berry, S. W. (1991). Evaluating meaningful auditory integration in profoundly hearing-impaired children. *American Journal of Otology, 12*(Suppl.), 144–150

Spencer, P. E. (2000). Every opportunity: A case study of hearing parents and their deaf child. In P. E. Spencer, C. J. Erting, & M. Marschark (Eds.), *The deaf child in the family and at school, Essays in honor of Kathryn P. Meadow-Orlans.* London: Lawrence Erlbaum Associates.

Starr, A., McPherson, D., Patterson, J., Luxford, W., Shannon, R., Sininger, Y., Tonokawa, L., & Waring, M. (1991). Absence of both auditory evoked potentials and auditory percepts dependent on time cues. *Brain, 114,* 1157–1180.

Starr, A., Picton, T. W., Sininger, Y. S., Hood, L. J., & Berlin, C. I. (1996). Auditory neuropathy. *Brain, 119,* 741–753.

Stinson, M. S., & Foster, F. (2000). Socialization of deaf children and youths in school. In P. E. Spencer, C. J. Erting, & M. Marschark (Eds.), *The deaf child in the family and at school, Essays in honor of Kathryn P. Meadow-Orlans.* London: Lawrence Erlbaum Associates.

Tye-Murray, N. (1998). *Foundations of aural rehabilitation.* San Diego: Singular Publishing Group.

Zeng, F. G., Oba, S., Garde, S., Sininger, Y., & Starr, A. (1999). Temporal and speech processing deficits in auditory neuropathy. *NeuroReport, 10,* 3429–3435.

Index

Vertigo, 129
Vestibular ocular reflex (VOR), 172
Vibration of tympanic membrane, 90
Visual audiometry (VRA) procedures,
     244
Visually supported spoken language,
     other methods of, 242–243

W

W-shaped bundle, 86
Wave II of ABR, 94
Wave V, 146
     preserved, 47
Word recognition, affecting, 8